Introduction to Motivational Interviewing for Mental Health Clinicians

A Practical Guide to Empowering Change in Mental Health Care

I0102949

Philip Jericho Townsend

ISBN: 978-1-7637425-1-2

Jstone Publishing

2nd Edition

Table of Contents

Preface

In the ever-evolving landscape of mental health care, clinicians continually seek effective tools and approaches to support their clients on the journey toward healing and self-discovery. Amidst the myriad therapeutic models available, one approach has steadily risen in prominence due to its unique combination of compassion, client autonomy, and practical effectiveness: Motivational Interviewing (MI). It is with great enthusiasm and a deep sense of responsibility that I present "**Introduction to Motivational Interviewing for Mental Health Clinicians**."

This book is born out of a dual intention. First, to demystify the principles and practices of MI for mental health professionals who are new to this approach, offering them a solid foundation from which to start. Second, to provide a refreshingly clear and practical guide for those who are familiar with MI but seek to deepen their understanding and refine their skills.

MI represents more than just a set of techniques; it embodies a philosophy of care that respects the inherent worth and potential of every individual. It aligns with the core values many of us hold dear in the mental health field: empathy, respect, collaboration, and empowerment. Through the pages of this book, I aim to convey not only the 'how' of MI but also the 'why'—the transformative power it holds for both clients and clinicians when practiced with fidelity and heart.

Drawing upon decades of research, clinical wisdom, and the collective experiences of MI practitioners worldwide, this book navigates the theoretical underpinnings, practical applications, and the nuanced dynamics of the MI process. From the foundational principles and techniques to advanced topics such as integrating MI with other therapeutic modalities and adapting it for diverse populations, each chapter is designed to be both informative and engaging.

The journey of writing this book has been one of profound learning and reaffirmation of my commitment to MI. It has reinforced my belief in the capacity for change that resides within each individual and the pivotal role of therapeutic relationships in unlocking this potential.

To the mental health clinicians who hold this book in their hands: my hope is that it serves as a valuable companion in your professional journey. It will inspire you to embrace MI's spirit, enhance your practice, and enrich the lives of those you serve. Whether you are at the beginning of your MI journey or looking to deepen your practice, I invite you to engage with this material with curiosity, openness, and a willingness to explore the transformative potential of Motivational Interviewing.

With gratitude and optimism for the path ahead,

Philip Jericho Townsend

Introduction

Introduction to Motivational Interviewing (MI) and Its Significance in Mental Health Care

Motivational Interviewing (MI) is a client-centered, directive method of communication with particular application in the field of mental health for eliciting behavior change by helping clients to explore and resolve ambivalence. Developed in the 1980s by clinical psychologists William R. Miller and Stephen Rollnick, MI has since evolved into a fundamental approach in various areas of healthcare, substance abuse treatment, and counseling. At its core, MI is predicated on the concept of collaborative conversation to strengthen an individual's own motivation and commitment to change.

The Spirit of MI

The essence of MI lies in its spirit, a way of being with clients that is characterized by respect, curiosity, and a kind of partnership that honors the client's expertise on their own life. It is defined by four key elements:

1. **Partnership**: MI is a collaborative approach, contrasting with traditional expert/patient dynamics. It emphasizes working together to explore and resolve ambivalence.

2. **Acceptance**: Practitioners of MI express acceptance towards their clients, recognizing and affirming their worth, potential, and strengths.

3. **Compassion**: A commitment to seek the best for the client, underpinning all MI interactions.

4. **Evocation**: MI practitioners strive to evoke the client's own motivations for change rather than imposing external motivations.

Significance in Mental Health Care

MI addresses a critical component often encountered in mental health care: the ambivalence towards change. Whether it's adopting healthier habits, overcoming substance use, or engaging in treatment for mental health disorders, clients often find themselves in two minds about making a change. MI helps in navigating this ambivalence, not through persuasion or coercion, but by facilitating an environment where clients can articulate their reasons for change in a safe and non-judgmental space.

Key Principles of MI

MI is guided by several principles that shape the interaction between clinician and client:

- **Express empathy** through reflective listening.

- **Develop discrepancy** between the client's current behaviors and their broader goals or values.

- **Avoid argumentation**, as confrontation tends to increase resistance.

- **Roll with resistance** by accepting it and exploring its sources, rather than opposing it directly.

- **Support self-efficacy** and optimism for change.

Impact on Mental Health Outcomes

Research and practice have shown that MI can significantly impact mental health outcomes. It has been effective in treating a wide range of issues, including substance abuse, depression, anxiety, and eating disorders, among others. MI's non-confrontational, empathetic approach reduces resistance and enhances client engagement, making it an invaluable tool in the mental health professional's repertoire.

In mental health care, MI's significance cannot be overstated. It empowers clients, respects their autonomy, and supports them in navigating the complex process of change. By focusing on the client's own motivations and strengths, MI facilitates a deeper engagement with the therapeutic process and promotes lasting change. This introduction to MI sets the stage for understanding how this approach can be integrated into practice, offering mental health clinicians a powerful method to enhance therapeutic outcomes and support clients on their journey towards well-being.

Overview of the Book's Unique Gamified and Interactive Approach

"Motivational Interviewing for Mental Health Clinicians Made Easy" is designed to revolutionize the way mental health professionals learn and apply the principles and techniques of Motivational Interviewing (MI). By incorporating a unique gamified and interactive approach, this book transcends traditional learning methods, engaging readers in an immersive experience that not only teaches but also entertains and challenges. This innovative approach aims to enhance learning retention, improve skill application in real-world settings, and make the journey of mastering MI both enjoyable and effective.

Interactive Case Studies

At the heart of the book's approach are the interactive case studies, which are carefully crafted narratives that simulate real-life scenarios clinicians might encounter in their practice. These case studies are not just stories to read; they are challenges to engage with. Readers are presented with choices at critical junctures, each leading to different outcomes based on the principles of MI. This interactive element allows readers to experiment with various approaches, learn from mistakes, and see the consequences of their choices in a controlled, risk-free environment.

Gamified Learning Elements

The gamification of learning elements introduces a competitive and rewarding aspect to mastering MI. Readers can earn points, badges, or achievements for successfully navigating case studies, demonstrating understanding of MI concepts, and applying skills effectively. This system not only motivates learners to progress through the book but also provides tangible milestones of their learning journey. Challenges and leaderboards can foster a community of practice among readers, encouraging sharing of insights, strategies, and experiences.

Real-time Feedback Mechanisms

A crucial component of the book's approach is the provision of real-time feedback. As readers make choices within the interactive case studies, immediate feedback is provided, highlighting the strengths and weaknesses of each decision in the context of MI principles. This feedback is designed to be constructive, offering explanations and suggestions for improvement, thereby facilitating a deeper understanding of MI techniques and how they can be applied in various situations.

Personal Progress Tracker

To complement the interactive and gamified elements, the book includes access to a personal progress tracker. This tool allows readers to monitor their advancement through the book, track the development of their MI skills, and reflect on learning outcomes. It serves as a personalized dashboard, showcasing achievements, areas for growth, and recommendations for further practice.

Community Challenges and Peer Learning

The book encourages active participation in community challenges, where readers can submit their responses to case studies, share their approaches to difficult conversations, and receive feedback from peers and experts. This element of peer learning and community support adds a dynamic layer to the educational experience, promoting a collaborative environment where mental health clinicians can learn from each other and grow together.

Conclusion

By integrating these innovative learning methods, "Motivational Interviewing for Mental Health Clinicians Made Easy" offers a comprehensive, engaging, and effective way to master MI. The gamified and interactive approach not only makes learning more enjoyable but also more impactful, equipping mental health professionals with the skills and confidence to apply MI principles in their practice and ultimately enhance therapeutic outcomes for their clients.

How to Use This Book: Navigating the Simulations, Case Studies, and Feedback Mechanisms

"Motivational Interviewing for Mental Health Clinicians Made Easy" is designed to be an immersive learning experience, leveraging simulations, interactive case studies, and real-time feedback to deepen your understanding and application of Motivational Interviewing (MI) techniques. This section provides a guide on how to navigate these components effectively, ensuring you make the most of what this innovative book has to offer.

Starting with the Basics

- **Read the foundational chapters first**: Before diving into the interactive elements, familiarize yourself with the fundamental concepts of MI outlined in the initial chapters. This foundational knowledge will enhance your engagement with the simulations and case studies.

Engaging with Interactive Case Studies

- **Choose your path**: Each case study presents you with choices that mimic real-life decisions you might make as a clinician. These decision points are crucial for learning; select the option you believe best aligns with MI principles.

- **Reflect on outcomes**: After making a choice, you'll see the outcome of your decision. Take time to reflect on how the result aligns with the goals of MI and what it teaches about client interaction.

Utilizing Real-time Feedback

- **Embrace feedback as a learning tool**: As you navigate through the case studies, you'll receive immediate feedback on your choices. This feedback is designed to highlight both the strengths and weaknesses of your decisions, offering insights into how you can more effectively apply MI techniques.

- **Iterative learning**: Don't be afraid to make mistakes. The feedback mechanism is there to guide your learning process. If a particular scenario doesn't go as planned, consider what the feedback suggests and how you might approach a similar situation differently in the future.

Advancing through Gamified Learning Elements

- **Track your progress**: Use the gamified elements such as points, badges, or achievements to monitor your progression through the book. These elements are designed to motivate and provide a tangible sense of accomplishment as you master MI skills.

- **Engage in community challenges**: Participate in challenges to test your skills against those of other readers. These activities are opportunities for peer learning and can offer new perspectives on applying MI.

Making the Most of the Personal Progress Tracker

- **Set up your tracker**: Early in the book, you'll be introduced to the personal progress tracker. Take the time to set it up and familiarize yourself with its features.

- **Regularly review your progress**: Refer back to your tracker regularly to assess your skill development, reflect on learning outcomes, and identify areas where further practice or revision might be beneficial.

- **Reflect on your learning**: Use the tracker as a reflective tool. It's not just about tracking progress; it's also about considering how you can apply what you've learned in your professional practice.

Participating in the Community

- **Engage with the community**: The book's approach is not just about individual learning; it's also about learning from and with others. Engage with the community through shared challenges, discussion forums, or peer feedback sessions to enrich your learning experience.

Continuous Practice and Application

- **Apply what you learn**: The ultimate goal of this book is to enhance your MI skills in real-world settings. Look for opportunities to apply techniques in your professional practice and reflect on these experiences in your progress tracker.

Conclusion

By actively engaging with the simulations, case studies, feedback mechanisms, and community challenges, you'll gain a deep, practical understanding of MI that goes beyond theoretical knowledge. This book is a tool for both learning and application; use it as a guide on your journey to becoming a more effective mental health clinician through the practice of Motivational Interviewing.

Chapter 1: Fundamentals of Motivational Interviewing

Definition and origins of MI
Definition

Motivational Interviewing (MI) is a client-centered, directive method of communication aimed at enhancing an individual's intrinsic motivation to change by exploring and resolving ambivalence. It is grounded in the concept of empowering clients to discover their own reasons and drive for making positive changes in their behavior, rather than being told what to do by the therapist. MI is characterized by its focus on collaboration between the therapist and client, evocation of the client's own motivations for change, and respect for the client's autonomy.

Origins

The origins of Motivational Interviewing can be traced back to the early 1980s, when Dr. William R. Miller, a clinical psychologist, introduced the approach in a seminal article published in 1983. Miller's work was initially inspired by his observations of the treatment of problem drinkers and the counterproductive effects of confrontational counseling styles. He noted that a more empathetic and supportive approach seemed to elicit a greater willingness to change among clients.

The development of MI was further advanced through collaboration with Dr. Stephen Rollnick, a clinical psychologist with a background in the treatment of addictions. Together, Miller and Rollnick refined MI into a more cohesive and comprehensive approach, emphasizing the therapeutic relationship as a key element in fostering change.

Their collaboration led to the publication of the first edition of "Motivational Interviewing: Preparing People to Change Addictive Behavior" in 1991, which laid the foundational principles and practices of MI.

Key Influences

The development of MI was influenced by several key psychological theories and practices, including:

- **Client-Centered Therapy**: Developed by Carl Rogers, this approach emphasizes empathy, unconditional positive regard, and congruence in the therapeutic relationship. MI adopts these principles, focusing on understanding the client's perspective and fostering a supportive environment for change.

- **Cognitive Dissonance Theory**: This theory suggests that people are motivated to change when they experience a discrepancy between their current behaviors and their personal values or goals. MI utilizes this concept by helping clients explore and resolve ambivalence toward change.

- **Self-Efficacy Theory**: Proposed by Albert Bandura, this theory highlights the importance of an individual's belief in their ability to succeed in specific situations. MI seeks to enhance clients' confidence in their ability to change by building on their strengths and past successes.

Evolution of MI

Since its inception, MI has evolved and expanded beyond its initial focus on addiction treatment to include applications in a wide range of behavioral health and medical settings. Its principles have been adapted for use in managing chronic health conditions, promoting healthy lifestyle changes, and addressing psychiatric disorders, among others.

The approach has also been enriched by ongoing research and the development of training methodologies that have helped to clarify and refine MI techniques, making it an evidence-based practice in the field of psychotherapy and counseling. Today, MI is recognized as a versatile and effective approach for facilitating behavioral change, respected for its empathetic, respectful, and client-centered nature.

As Motivational Interviewing (MI) continued to gain traction across various disciplines, its applications broadened significantly. Researchers and practitioners have explored its efficacy in contexts such as diabetes management, cardiovascular health, dietary changes, physical activity promotion, smoking cessation, and adherence to medication regimens. This expansion reflects MI's versatility and its adaptability to diverse client needs and settings.

Key Components of MI

Despite its broad applicability, the core components of MI have remained consistent, centered around its fundamental principles:

1. **Collaboration versus Confrontation**: MI is based on a partnership that respects the client's autonomy and perspective, contrasting sharply with approaches that confront or direct the client.

2. **Drawing Out Client's Motivations**: The focus is on evoking the client's own reasons for change, rather than imposing external motivations.

3. **Autonomy Support**: MI emphasizes the client's control over their decision-making process, supporting intrinsic motivation to change.

Training and Dissemination

The dissemination of MI has been facilitated through comprehensive training programs, certification processes, and the establishment of the Motivational Interviewing Network of Trainers (MINT) in 1997. MINT is an international organization committed to promoting high-quality MI practice and training. Through workshops, seminars, and mentoring, MI practitioners are equipped with the skills necessary to apply the approach effectively in their work.

Research and Evidence Base

The effectiveness of MI has been rigorously tested in numerous research studies across various fields. Meta-analyses and systematic reviews have generally supported MI's efficacy, particularly in short-term interventions and for behaviors that require a high degree of personal motivation to change. Research has also explored the mechanisms by which MI exerts its effects, including the importance of therapist empathy, the resolution of ambivalence, and the enhancement of self-efficacy.

Challenges and Criticisms

While widely adopted and supported by evidence, MI has faced challenges and criticisms. Some practitioners struggle with the balance between directive and nondirective components of MI, particularly in drawing out change talk without imposing direction. There has also been debate about the specific contexts in which MI is most effective, and how it compares to other interventions for long-term behavior change.

Future Directions

Looking forward, MI continues to evolve in response to new research findings and clinical experiences. Innovations in training, including the use of technology and virtual reality for skill development, are expanding the reach and impact of MI. Additionally, the integration of MI with other therapeutic approaches offers promising avenues for enhancing its effectiveness and applicability.

The continued exploration of MI's principles and practices, bolstered by a robust research agenda, ensures that MI remains a dynamic and vital approach within the mental health and medical fields. Its emphasis on empathy, respect, and collaboration aligns well with contemporary movements toward person-centered and recovery-oriented care, positioning MI as a key component of effective therapeutic practice for years to come.

Core principles and spirit of MI

Motivational Interviewing (MI) is like having a respectful and supportive conversation that helps people talk about their need for change and find their own motivation to make those changes. It's based on a few key principles and a certain spirit that guides these conversations.

Core Principles of MI

1. **Partnership**: This is about working together. Imagine a dance rather than a tug-of-war. The therapist and client are partners in this journey, collaborating and exploring ideas together.

2. **Acceptance**: This means respecting and valuing the client just as they are, understanding their worth, and recognizing their strengths and efforts.

3. **Compassion**: Every conversation is guided by a genuine desire to help and support the client's welfare and best interests.

4. **Evocation**: This is about drawing out the client's own thoughts and motivations for change, rather than telling them what to do. It's like helping someone find their own reasons to change, rather than giving them yours.

Spirit of MI

The spirit of MI is the overall attitude or way of being that encompasses these principles. It's about approaching conversations with kindness, curiosity, and a willingness to truly listen and understand the client's perspective. In MI, it's important to create a warm and supportive environment where clients feel comfortable exploring their ambivalence about change without feeling judged or pressured.

In simpler terms, MI is like a helpful and empathetic friend who listens carefully, understands your struggles, helps you find your own reasons to change, and supports you through the process, all without judging or pushing you.

The role of empathy and listening in MI

In Motivational Interviewing (MI), empathy and listening are super important, kind of like the superpowers of a good friend who's there for you when you need help. Here's why they matter so much:

Empathy in MI

- **Understanding Feelings**: Empathy is all about really getting how someone else is feeling. In MI, it means the therapist tries to understand the world from your point of view, not just hearing your words but feeling what you're feeling.

- **Creating a Safe Space**: When you know someone gets you, it feels safe to open up. This safety lets you talk about things that might be hard or scary to think about changing.

- **Building Trust**: Showing empathy helps build trust. When you feel understood, you're more likely to trust the therapist and believe they have your best interests at heart.

Listening in MI

- **Hearing Beyond Words**: Good listening in MI isn't just about waiting for your turn to speak. It's about really hearing what's being said, both the words and the feelings or doubts hidden underneath.

- **Reflecting and Clarifying**: By listening closely, a therapist can reflect back what you've said in a way that helps you see things more clearly or consider them in a new light. This can help you understand your own thoughts and feelings better.

- **Encouraging Exploration**: When someone listens to you really well, it encourages you to explore your thoughts and feelings more deeply. It can help you discover your own reasons for wanting to change.

Deepening Understanding

When therapists listen with empathy, they can help clients dig deeper into their own motivations and concerns. It's like gently peeling back layers to reveal what's really holding someone back or what truly motivates them. This deeper understanding can be the key to unlocking a person's readiness to change.

Reducing Resistance

Change is hard, and talking about change can sometimes make people defensive or resistant. Empathy and good listening can lower these defenses. When clients feel understood, not judged, they're more likely to open up and less likely to resist the process of change. It's like turning down the volume on fear and turning up the courage to look at things differently.

Strengthening Relationship

The relationship between the therapist and client is a big part of what makes MI work. Empathy and active listening are the building blocks of this relationship. They create a bond of trust and respect that makes it easier for clients to consider making changes. This relationship is not about one person fixing another; it's about working together to explore possibilities.

Facilitating Self-Discovery

One of the most powerful aspects of MI is helping clients come to their own realizations about change. Through empathetic listening, therapists can guide clients to voice their own reasons for change, which is often more motivating than being told why they should change. It's like helping someone find the map inside them that leads to where they want to go.

Encouraging Empowerment

Ultimately, empathy and listening in MI are about empowering clients. By truly hearing and understanding clients, therapists help them to see that they have the strength and ability to make changes. This empowerment is a crucial step toward lasting change because it comes from within the client, not imposed from the outside.

In simpler terms, think of empathy and listening in MI as the warm, supportive embrace that everyone needs when facing tough decisions or changes. They are the foundation for a journey of self-discovery, growth, and change, making it possible for clients to move forward with confidence and a sense of ownership over their decisions.

Ambivalence and behavior change

Understanding ambivalence in the context of behavior change is like recognizing that someone can have mixed feelings about making a change, even if that change is good for them. Imagine you're thinking about starting to exercise more. Part of you might be excited about getting fit and feeling healthier, but another part might dread the idea of waking up early to go for a run or giving up some free time.

Why Ambivalence is Normal

- **Two Minds**: It's normal to feel two ways about something because change is hard. It means leaving our comfort zone, which can feel scary or uncertain.

- **Comfort vs. Change**: Our brains like routines and the familiar. Even if part of us wants to change for the better, another part might resist because it feels safer or easier to stay the same.

Ambivalence in Behavior Change

- **The Tug of War**: When we talk about changing behavior, ambivalence is like an internal tug of war. One side pulls towards the benefits of changing, while the other side pulls back towards the comfort of staying the same.

- **Acknowledging Mixed Feelings**: Recognizing this tug of war is the first step. It's okay to have mixed feelings about change. Acknowledging them helps us understand what's holding us back and what could motivate us to move forward.

The Role of Ambivalence in Everyday Life

Imagine you're considering a major life decision, like changing jobs. Part of you is excited about the new opportunities and growth potential, while another part might fear the unknown or the possibility of not fitting in. This ambivalence isn't just indecision; it's a reflection of the complex, often conflicting feelings and thoughts we have about change. It shows up in big life decisions and small daily choices alike, influencing our behavior in profound ways.

Why Recognizing Ambivalence is Crucial

- **Self-Awareness**: Acknowledging ambivalence increases self-awareness. It helps you understand why you might be procrastinating or feeling stuck. This awareness is the first step toward meaningful change.

- **Reduces Guilt and Shame**: Understanding that ambivalence is normal can reduce feelings of guilt or shame that come from struggling with change. It's a reminder that you're human, and it's okay to have conflicting feelings.

How MI Turns Ambivalence into a Catalyst for Change

- **Creates a Safe Space for Exploration**: MI provides a non-judgmental space to explore these mixed feelings. By discussing ambivalence openly, individuals can start to understand their own motivations and concerns more clearly.

- **Encourages Looking at the Bigger Picture**: Through reflective listening and targeted questions, MI helps individuals consider the broader impact of their choices. What might they gain by making a change? What might they lose by staying the same? This can help clarify values and priorities.

- **Empowers the Individual**: Ultimately, MI shifts the focus from ambivalence as a barrier to ambivalence as a source of insight. It empowers individuals to use their mixed feelings as a tool for understanding what they really want and for making decisions that align with their values and goals.

How MI Helps with Ambivalence

Motivational Interviewing (MI) helps by:

- **Listening**: MI involves listening to all the mixed feelings without judgment. This helps people feel understood and safe to explore their feelings more deeply.

- **Exploring Both Sides**: It encourages talking about both the good things about changing and the hard parts. This can help make sense of the tug of war and start to tip the balance towards change.

- **Finding Personal Reasons**: MI helps people discover their own, personal reasons for wanting to change, which is often more powerful than someone else telling them why they should change.

Moving Forward with Ambivalence

Understanding and working through ambivalence is not about eliminating these mixed feelings; it's about learning to navigate them more effectively. It's like being at a crossroads and recognizing that each path has its pros and cons. MI doesn't push you down a path; instead, it offers a map and a compass, helping you to chart your own course based on a deeper understanding of your motivations and fears.

Conclusion

In simple terms, ambivalence is a natural part of the human experience, especially when it comes to making changes. Recognizing and exploring these mixed feelings can be a powerful step towards growth. Motivational Interviewing serves as a supportive guide in this process, turning ambivalence from a stumbling block into a stepping stone towards positive change. It's about harnessing the energy from those conflicting feelings to propel yourself forward in a direction that feels right for you.

Chapter 2: Engaging the Client

Techniques for establishing rapport and trust.

Building rapport and trust is like making a new friend. It's about creating a comfortable and safe space where both people feel understood and respected. When it comes to therapy or counseling, here are some simple ways therapists can build that kind of relationship with their clients:

1. Smile and Use a Warm Tone

Think of how you feel when someone greets you with a genuine smile and speaks in a friendly tone. It makes you feel welcome and valued, right? Therapists start building trust from the first hello, using their body language and voice to show they're approachable and caring.

2. Listen More Than You Talk

Everyone wants to feel heard. When therapists listen more than they talk, it sends a message that the client's thoughts and feelings matter. It's like saying, "I'm here for you, and I want to understand your world."

3. Reflect Back What You Hear

Imagine telling someone about your day, and they repeat back the key points, showing they really get it. That's what therapists do. They mirror back what clients say, showing they're listening closely and truly understand.

4. Show Genuine Interest

Just like getting to know a friend, therapists show they care by being curious about the client's life, asking thoughtful questions without being nosy or judgmental. It's about wanting to know the person, not just the problem.

5. Be Consistent and Reliable

Trust builds over time when therapists are consistent in their actions and words. Showing up on time, keeping promises, and staying steady through ups and downs tells clients they can count on their therapist.

6. Share a Little About Yourself (When Appropriate)

Sometimes, therapists might share a tiny bit about their own experiences or feelings, if it helps the client feel less alone or more understood. But it's always done carefully, making sure it's for the client's benefit, not the therapist's.

7. Acknowledge and Respect Boundaries

Good friends understand and respect each other's boundaries. Similarly, therapists make it clear they respect clients' privacy and limits, which makes clients feel safe and protected.

8. Be Patient and Non-Judgmental

Building a friendship doesn't happen overnight, and neither does building a therapeutic relationship. Therapists show patience, letting the relationship develop at the client's pace, without judging or pushing.

9. Use Humor Wisely

Just like in any good friendship, a well-placed joke or light-hearted comment can break the ice and make the room feel warmer. When a therapist uses humor appropriately, it can help to relieve tension and show their human side, making clients feel more at ease.

10. Validate Their Feelings

When clients share their feelings, therapists can validate them by acknowledging those emotions as real and significant. It's like saying, "It makes sense you feel that way," which helps clients feel understood and accepted.

11. Offer Encouragement

Encouragement goes a long way. When therapists highlight a client's strengths or progress, no matter how small, it boosts their confidence and reinforces the trust in the therapeutic relationship. It's like cheering on a friend who's working towards a goal.

12. Maintain Confidentiality

One of the cornerstones of trust in therapy is confidentiality. Clients need to know that what they share in therapy stays in therapy (except in cases where there's a risk of harm). It's like having a vault where clients can safely store their most personal thoughts and feelings.

13. Create a Collaborative Environment

Rapport and trust flourish in an environment where clients feel they're working together with their therapist, not just being told what to do. By setting goals together and involving the client in decisions about their treatment, therapists foster a sense of partnership.

14. Practice Empathy Actively

Active empathy means not just understanding and sharing someone's feelings but also conveying that empathy back to the client. It's an active process of showing, "I'm with you in this." It helps clients feel deeply seen and supported.

15. Be Honest and Transparent

Honesty and transparency about the therapy process can significantly enhance trust. When therapists are clear about what clients can expect, including the limitations and potential challenges of therapy, it builds a foundation of trust and realistic expectations.

16. Adapt Your Approach

Just like every friend is unique, every client is different. Therapists show their respect and commitment by adapting their approach to fit the individual needs and comfort levels of each client, whether it's adjusting the pace of sessions or being mindful of cultural backgrounds.

Conclusion

Building rapport and trust in therapy is about making a genuine connection. It involves listening, understanding, respecting, and walking alongside the client on their journey. These techniques aren't just strategies; they're manifestations of a therapist's genuine care and commitment to their client's well-being. Just like in any meaningful relationship, it's about creating a space where the client feels valued, understood, and supported every step of the way.

The art of reflective listening.

Reflective listening is like being a mirror for someone's words and feelings. Imagine someone tells you about their day, and you carefully listen, then respond in a way that shows you really get what they're saying and how they're feeling.Reflective listening isn't just about the mechanics of mirroring back what someone says; it's about engaging with the whole person—their words, emotions, and even what they're not saying directly. That's reflective listening in a nutshell. Here's how it works in simple terms:

Paying Close Attention

First, you need to really listen to what the other person is saying, without thinking about what you're going to say next or getting distracted by your own thoughts. It's like tuning into a radio station where the only thing playing is the other person's words and feelings.

Mirroring Back

After you've listened, you reflect or mirror back what you've heard. But you don't just repeat their words like a parrot. Instead, you might rephrase what they said in your own words, showing that you're trying to understand their perspective. It's like saying, "So, it sounds like you're feeling really overwhelmed because of all the work you have to do."

Checking for Understanding

Sometimes, to make sure you've got it right, you might ask a question or make a statement that gives the other person a chance to correct you if you've misunderstood. It's a bit like guessing the end of a story and then asking, "Is that right?" This helps the person feel really heard and understood.

Showing Empathy

Reflective listening is also about connecting with how the other person feels about what they're saying. You acknowledge their emotions, which shows empathy. For example, you might say, "It sounds like that was a really tough decision for you," which shows you're not just hearing the words but also feeling the weight of their experience.

Listen for the Unspoken

People don't always say everything they're feeling or thinking directly. Sometimes, what's not said is as important as what is. Pay attention to tone of voice, pauses, and body language. Reflecting back on these unspoken messages can be powerful, like saying, "You seem hesitant, is there something you're unsure about?" This shows you're truly attentive to their whole message.

Validate Emotions

When you recognize and name someone's emotions as you reflect back, it validates their feelings. This can be incredibly reassuring and can make the person feel safe and supported. For example, "It sounds like you're really passionate about this project, and it's frustrating when others don't see its value." This validation helps build emotional trust.

Encourage Exploration

By reflecting back in a way that opens up more depth, you encourage the other person to explore their thoughts and feelings more deeply. Phrases like, "What do you think led you to feel this way?" invite further reflection and conversation. It's like gently helping someone unpack a suitcase filled with their thoughts and feelings.

Use Silence Wisely

Silence can be a powerful tool in reflective listening. After reflecting back, giving the other person space to respond or continue can be very meaningful. It shows that you're patient and willing to be there with them, in the moment, as they process their thoughts and feelings.

Reflective Listening in Difficult Conversations

Reflective listening becomes even more crucial during difficult or sensitive conversations. Here, the aim is to reduce defensiveness and open up dialogue. For instance, in a conflict, reflecting back the other person's viewpoint before sharing your own can help de-escalate tension and lead to a more productive discussion.

Practice Makes Perfect

Becoming skilled at reflective listening takes practice. It's about tuning in to the other person with your full attention, which can be challenging in a world full of distractions. Regularly practicing reflective listening, even in everyday conversations, can greatly enhance your ability to connect with others.

Why It's Powerful

When you listen reflectively, you do a few important things:

- **You make the other person feel heard and understood**, which can be incredibly validating and comforting.

- **You help clarify thoughts and feelings**, both for yourself and the other person, which can sometimes make a confusing situation a bit clearer.

- **You build a stronger connection** with the other person, as they're likely to feel more comfortable sharing with someone who really listens and understands.

In essence, the art of reflective listening is about being fully present, tuning into the other person's experience, and responding in a way that makes them feel valued and understood. It's a simple but powerful way to enhance communication and deepen relationships.

Identifying and eliciting change talk.

Identifying and eliciting change talk is like being a detective who's searching for clues that someone is thinking about making a change. Change talk means any kind of speech that shows a person is considering changing a behavior, attitude, or situation. Here's how it works, explained in a simple, easy-to-understand way:

What is Change Talk?

Imagine a friend saying, "I really should start eating healthier," or, "I feel better when I exercise." These statements are "change talk" because they show your friend is thinking about making a change for the better. It's like little hints that they're ready to move in a positive direction, even if they're not 100% there yet.

Why is Identifying Change Talk Important?

Finding and encouraging change talk is super important because:

- It's like watering a plant. The more you water it (encourage change talk), the more it grows (the more the person starts believing in the possibility of change).

- It helps you understand what motivates someone and what's holding them back, making it easier to support them in the right way.

How to Identify Change Talk

Change talk can come in different flavors, like:

- **Desire to change**: "I want to..."

- **Ability to change**: "I can..."

- **Reasons to change**: "It would be good if..."

- **Need to change**: "I need to..."

- **Commitment to change**: "I will..."

- **Taking steps toward change**: "I've started to..."

Listen for these clues in conversations. They're signs that someone is warming up to the idea of change.

How to Elicit Change Talk

1. **Ask Open-Ended Questions**: These are questions that can't be answered with a simple "yes" or "no." They encourage people to talk more about their feelings and thoughts. For example, "What makes you think you want to start exercising?"

2. **Use Reflective Listening**: This means listening closely to what someone says and then reflecting it back to them in

your own words. It shows you understand and encourages them to keep talking. If someone says, "I feel so much better when I'm not smoking," you might respond, "So, not smoking makes you feel healthier?"

3. **Highlight the Positives**: Point out the good things that could come from making a change. If someone's unsure about quitting smoking, you might say, "What are some benefits you might see if you decided to quit?"

4. **Explore Ambivalence**: Talk about the mixed feelings they might have. It's okay to discuss why they're hesitant or what's tough about making a change. Asking, "What's the hardest part about the idea of quitting?" can open up a lot of insights.

5. **Encourage with Affirmations**: Positive feedback can boost someone's confidence. Simple affirmations like, "You've made big changes before; I believe you can do this too," can be very motivating.

Building on the idea of identifying and eliciting change talk, let's delve deeper into how you can further nurture and strengthen this inclination towards change. Think of change talk as a seed that, when properly watered and cared for, can grow into a strong tree of transformation. Here's how to keep that growth going:

Expand on the Positives

When someone expresses even a tiny bit of interest in changing, latch onto it and help them expand that thought. Ask them to imagine the future and describe what it would look like if they made the change. Questions like, "How would your life be different if you made this change?" help them visualize the benefits and solidify their desire to change.

Link Changes to Personal Values

People are more motivated to change when they see how the change aligns with their personal values or important life goals. If someone values being a good parent, and they're thinking about quitting smoking, you might discuss how this change supports their value of family health and being a role model for their children. Asking, "How does making this change reflect who you are or who you want to be?" can make the change feel more meaningful.

Normalize Ambivalence

It's important to let the person know it's normal to feel conflicted about change. This can reduce their inner tension and make the process feel more manageable. Say something like, "Most people find themselves feeling two ways about change. It's completely normal." This reassurance can make them feel understood and less alone in their struggle.

Strengthen Commitment Language

When you hear someone moving from "I might" to "I will," recognize and reinforce this stronger language of commitment. Congratulate them on this shift and explore what made them more certain. Questions like, "What helped you decide?" can reinforce their commitment and help them articulate their motivation more clearly.

Celebrate Small Wins

Change is often a slow process with ups and downs. Celebrating small wins and steps in the right direction can build momentum. If someone has cut down on smoking, for example, acknowledge their effort and discuss how this step brings them closer to their goal. This encouragement can boost their confidence to keep going.

Use Scaling Questions

Scaling questions can help someone evaluate their readiness, confidence, and importance of making a change on a scale from 1 to 10. For instance, "On a scale from 1 to 10, how important is it for you to make this change?" Follow-up questions can explore what it would take to move from a lower number to a higher one, helping to elicit more change talk.

Reflect on Past Successes

Discussing past successes in making changes, even if they're unrelated, can increase confidence. Ask, "Can you tell me about a time when you successfully made a change in your life? What worked for you then?" This conversation can help them see their own capacity for change and apply lessons from past experiences.

Conclusion

Identifying and eliciting change talk is all about listening for hints that someone wants to make a change, then encouraging them to talk more about it. It's like being a supportive friend who helps them see their own reasons and abilities to make positive changes. By doing this, you help them water their own plant of change, so it grows strong and healthy.

Case Study Simulation 1: Engaging a Hesitant Client

Background: Alex is a 35-year-old who has been referred for counseling by their primary care doctor due to concerns about stress and anxiety. Alex has never been to therapy before and is skeptical about its benefits. They have a busy work life and are unsure about dedicating time for therapy. Alex shows up for the first session but sits with arms crossed and appears guarded.

Objective: Your goal is to engage Alex, making them feel comfortable, understood, and open to the process of therapy.

Step 1: Establishing Rapport

- **Approach:** Start by creating a welcoming environment. Smile, introduce yourself warmly, and thank Alex for coming in. Acknowledge that making the decision to attend therapy can be tough and commend their willingness to show up.

- **Your Move:** "Alex, I'm really glad you're here today. I know coming in can feel like a big step, especially if it's your first time seeking therapy. Let's take this at your own pace. What brought you in today?"

Step 2: Reflective Listening

- **Scenario:** Alex shares that they've been feeling overwhelmed at work and losing sleep but quickly adds that they're not sure talking about problems actually helps.

- **Your Move:** Reflect back Alex's feelings and validate their skepticism. "It sounds like things have been really overwhelming for you, and it's affecting your sleep. It's completely understandable to question how talking about these problems might help. Many people feel that way initially. Can you tell me a bit more about what's been going on at work?"

Step 3: Normalize Ambivalence

- **Scenario:** Alex admits feeling torn between wanting to manage everything alone and acknowledging they might need help.

- **Your Move:** Normalize this ambivalence and connect it to a common human experience. "Feeling torn between wanting to handle things on your own and recognizing when it's time to seek help is a common experience. It shows a lot of self-awareness and strength. How do you feel about exploring these feelings together?"

Step 4: Elicit Change Talk

- **Scenario:** As the conversation progresses, Alex mentions a desire for things to be different but quickly downplays their ability to change.

- **Your Move:** Seize the moment to focus on Alex's desire for change. Ask open-ended questions to explore this further and encourage them to consider their strengths. "You mentioned wanting things to be different. What changes would you like to see in your life? What do you think are your strengths that can help you through this process?"

Step 5: Build Confidence

- **Scenario:** Alex expresses doubt about their ability to cope with stress and make meaningful changes.

- **Your Move:** Highlight Alex's step of coming to therapy as a sign of strength and readiness for change. Offer reassurance about the process. "Coming here today was a significant step towards managing your stress better. It shows you're ready to explore ways to feel better. Together, we can work on strategies that fit your life and help you move towards the changes you're hoping for."

Conclusion:

- Wrap up the session by summarizing key points discussed, affirming Alex's feelings and strengths, and setting a tentative goal for the next session. Encourage Alex to reflect on what they hope to achieve through therapy.

- **Your Closing Move:** "Today, we've started a valuable conversation about what you're experiencing and your mixed feelings about therapy. I'm here to support you through this journey. For our next session, let's think about one small change you feel ready to explore. How does that sound?"

This simulation aims to demonstrate how using empathy, validation, and strategic questioning can engage a hesitant client, making them feel heard, understood, and more open to the therapeutic process.

Case Study Simulation 2: Building Confidence in a Doubtful Client

Background: Jordan is a 28-year-old graphic designer who struggles with self-confidence and imposter syndrome, especially at work. Despite receiving positive feedback and recognition for their talent, Jordan feels like they don't truly belong in their field and fears being exposed as a fraud. They've started therapy to address these feelings but remain skeptical about their ability to overcome these doubts.

Objective: Your goal is to help Jordan build confidence and start to challenge their imposter syndrome through empathetic engagement and strategic exploration.

Step 1: Validate Feelings

- **Approach:** Begin by acknowledging Jordan's courage in seeking help and validate their feelings of doubt. Emphasize that imposter syndrome is common among high achievers.

- **Your Move:** "Jordan, it's great that you've decided to tackle these feelings head-on. Many talented individuals feel just as you do, questioning their success. It's a testament to your strength that you're here, ready to work through these doubts."

Step 2: Explore the Origin

- **Scenario:** Jordan shares that they've always felt the need to be perfect, stemming from high expectations in their family. They fear making mistakes and often overwork to prevent failure.

- **Your Move:** Use reflective listening to delve deeper into Jordan's experiences. "It sounds like the pressure to be perfect has been a significant weight on your shoulders, leading you to work even harder. How do you think these expectations have shaped your feelings of belonging in your career?"

Step 3: Identify Strengths and Successes

- **Scenario:** Jordan struggles to acknowledge their accomplishments, attributing success to luck rather than skill.

- **Your Move:** Encourage Jordan to list their achievements, no matter how small, and explore the skills and efforts that led to those successes. "Let's take a moment to look at some of your achievements. Can you think of one project you're proud of? What skills did you use to complete it? How does recognizing those skills challenge the idea that your success is just due to luck?"

Step 4: Challenge Negative Beliefs

- **Scenario:** Jordan expresses a pervasive belief that they are not as competent as others think.

- **Your Move:** Engage Jordan in examining the evidence for and against this belief. Introduce the concept of cognitive distortions and how they can skew self-perception. "When you feel like you're not competent, what specific thoughts come to mind? Let's look at those thoughts and the evidence supporting them. Could there be another way to view your skills and contributions?"

Step 5: Develop Coping Strategies

- **Scenario:** Jordan is open to change but unsure how to start feeling more confident.

- **Your Move:** Collaboratively develop coping strategies to deal with moments of doubt. This could include mindfulness exercises, keeping a success journal, or practicing assertive communication. "Building confidence is a process, and there are strategies we can use to help. For instance, keeping a journal of your successes might remind you of your capabilities. How do you feel about trying something like that?"

Conclusion:

- Summarize the session's key insights, reinforcing Jordan's willingness to challenge their imposter syndrome and highlighting any progress made. Set a goal for the next session based on the coping strategies discussed.

- **Your Closing Move:** "Today, we've started to uncover the roots of your feelings of doubt and looked at ways to build your confidence. Reflecting on your achievements and the effort behind them is a powerful step forward. For our next meeting, let's focus on one strategy you'd like to implement. How does that sound to you?"

This case study simulation aims to demonstrate the importance of empathetic listening, validation, and active engagement in helping clients like Jordan confront and manage feelings of self-doubt and imposter syndrome, setting the stage for meaningful personal growth and change.

Case Study Simulation 3: Navigating Grief with a Mourning Client

Background: Sam is a 42-year-old who recently lost a close family member. They have been struggling with intense grief, which has impacted their daily functioning and relationships. Sam decided to seek therapy to find ways to cope with their loss but feels stuck in their sorrow.

Objective: Your goal is to help Sam navigate their grief, providing support and strategies to manage their emotions and begin the healing process.

The Session Begins

Therapist: "Sam, I want to thank you for coming in today. I know that talking about your loss can be incredibly hard, but I'm here to support you through this. Can you tell me a little about your loved one and what you're going through?"

Sam: "It's been really tough... I miss them every day. Sometimes, it feels like I'm just going through the motions of life without really living. I'm not sure how to move past this."

Therapist: "It sounds like you're experiencing a deep sense of loss and emptiness. Grieving can certainly make us feel like we're stuck in a fog. It's important to acknowledge these feelings and not rush yourself through the grieving process. What are some moments in your day when you feel their absence the most?"

Sam: "Mealtimes are the hardest. We used to cook together. Now, I barely have the appetite to eat, let alone cook."

Therapist: "Mealtimes have become a reminder of your loss and the shared moments you cherished. It's understandable how this can affect your appetite and enjoyment of food. Have you thought about starting a small ritual during mealtimes that honors their memory?"

Sam: "I haven't, but I like the idea. Maybe I could cook their favorite dish once a week."

Therapist: "That sounds like a beautiful way to remember and celebrate their life. It's okay if it feels bittersweet at first. Engaging in meaningful activities can be a step toward healing. How do you feel about incorporating this into your week?"

Sam: "I think it could help. It feels like a way to keep them close."

Therapist: "Absolutely, keeping their memory alive through actions that were significant to both of you can be very therapeutic. It's also okay to have days where you don't feel up to it. Healing isn't linear, and it's important to be gentle with yourself. What other support do you have around you during this time?"

Sam: "I have friends who've been reaching out, but I often don't know what to say to them."

Therapist: "It can be challenging to communicate your needs when you're grieving. Sometimes, letting your friends know that you appreciate their presence, even if you're not ready to talk, can be enough. How would you feel about letting them in just a little, maybe by spending time together without the pressure of having to talk about your loss?"

Sam: "That might be good. I do miss being around them."

Therapist: "Reconnecting with your support network can be a source of comfort. Remember, it's okay to set boundaries around these interactions to protect your emotional space. For our next session, let's talk about how this week went, focusing on the cooking ritual and any interactions with your friends. How does that sound?"

Sam: "It sounds like a plan. Thank you."

Therapist: "Of course, Sam. I'm here for you. This journey through grief is yours, and I'll walk alongside you at your pace."

Conclusion:

This conversation showcases the therapist's use of empathy, validation, and gentle guidance to help Sam begin to navigate their grief. By suggesting tangible actions, like cooking a loved one's favorite dish and reconnecting with friends, the therapist provides Sam with strategies to cope with their loss while acknowledging the uniqueness of their grieving process.

Chapter 3: Focusing the Conversation

Guiding the conversation towards goals.

Guiding a conversation towards goals is a bit like being a gentle guide on a hiking trail. You have a map (the goal) and you're walking alongside someone, helping them choose the path that gets them to where they want to go. Here's how you can do this in simple steps:

1. Know the Destination

First, you need to know what the goal or destination is. This means understanding what the other person wants to achieve from the conversation. Ask questions like, "What do you hope to get out of our talk today?" This sets the direction for your journey together.

2. Keep the Path Clear

Imagine walking through a forest; the path can sometimes get cluttered with branches or rocks. In conversations, these are distractions or off-topic subjects. Gently steer the conversation back if it starts to wander off the path. You can say, "That's an interesting point, but let's focus on what we said we'd talk about."

3. Use Signposts

As you're guiding someone, it's helpful to point out landmarks or signposts along the way. In conversations, these are key points or milestones related to their goal. For example, if someone wants to talk about improving their time management, you might discuss specific strategies like making a to-do list or setting priorities.

4. Encourage Exploration

Sometimes, the person you're talking with might not be sure which path to take. Encourage them to explore different options by asking open-ended questions like, "What have you tried before?" or "What do you think might work best for you?" This helps them think through their options and decide on the best path forward.

5. Offer Support, Not Direction

Imagine you're walking behind them with a flashlight, illuminating the path, rather than leading them by the hand. Offer support and suggestions, but let them make the final decisions. This could look like saying, "Some people find it helpful to start small, like focusing on one task at a time. What do you think about trying that?"

6. Celebrate Progress

Every step forward, no matter how small, is progress. Acknowledge and celebrate these moments. "You've done a great job identifying what's been holding you back. How do you feel about the progress we've made today?" This builds confidence and motivation.

7. Adjust the Route as Needed

Sometimes, you'll find that the initial goal needs to be adjusted. Maybe there's a better path to take. It's okay to change direction based on new information or insights. "Now that we've talked about this more, do you still feel that's the right goal, or do you want to explore a different direction?"

8. Practice Active Listening

Active listening is essential. This means giving your full attention, nodding, making eye contact, and occasionally summarizing what the other person has said to show you understand. This technique ensures the speaker feels heard and valued, which can make them more open to exploring their goals and how to achieve them.

9. Use Positive Reinforcement

Everyone responds well to positive reinforcement. When the person you're talking to makes a valid point or takes a step toward their goal, acknowledge it with positive feedback. This could be as simple as saying, "That's a really good insight," or "I think that's a great step forward." This encouragement can boost their confidence and motivation.

10. Incorporate Visualization

Sometimes, helping someone visualize their goal or the steps needed to get there can be incredibly powerful. Ask them to imagine what achieving their goal would look and feel like. This can help make the goal more tangible and attainable in their mind, increasing their motivation to pursue it.

11. Set Small, Achievable Targets

Big goals can be overwhelming. Break them down into smaller, more manageable targets. This approach makes progress seem more achievable and less daunting. For example, if the goal is to get more organized, start with organizing one small area or aspect of life before tackling bigger ones.

12. Emphasize the Journey, Not Just the Destination

Remind them that achieving goals is often about the journey as much as the destination. The skills learned and the growth experienced along the way are just as valuable as reaching the goal itself. This perspective can help maintain motivation, especially when progress seems slow.

13. Create a Safe Space for Failure

It's important to discuss and normalize the possibility of setbacks or failures as part of the process. Encourage a mindset that views these not as failures but as learning opportunities. This can help reduce fear of failure and make the journey towards the goal less intimidating.

14. Develop a Follow-up Plan

Establish a way to check in on progress towards the goal. This could be a follow-up conversation, a written plan, or another form of accountability. Knowing there's a plan to revisit and assess progress can help keep the goal in focus and provide an opportunity for reassessment and adjustment if needed.

15. Cultivate Patience and Persistence

Encourage patience and persistence, reminding them that progress towards significant goals often takes time. Celebrate the persistence it takes to keep moving forward, even when progress is slow. This can help sustain motivation over the long term.

Conclusion

Guiding a conversation towards goals is all about understanding what the person wants to achieve, keeping the conversation focused, encouraging exploration of options, offering support, celebrating progress, and being flexible about the route you take. It's a collaborative journey where you help illuminate the path, but they choose the steps they take.

Recognizing and reinforcing client strengths.

Recognizing and reinforcing client strengths is like being a treasure hunter who helps people discover the gold hidden within themselves. Everyone has strengths and talents, but sometimes they're buried under doubts, fears, or tough times. Here's how this treasure hunt works in simple terms:

Spotting the Gold

First, you need to be really good at spotting those shiny bits of gold—the strengths. This means paying close attention to what someone is good at, even if they don't see it themselves. It could be their kindness, how they solve problems, or their creativity. It's like noticing someone is really good at finding their way when you're lost, even if they've never thought of themselves as a good navigator.

Shining a Light on It

Once you spot a strength, you shine a light on it so the person can see it too. You might say, "I've noticed you're really great at listening to your friends when they have problems. That's a special strength." It's like pointing out to someone that they have a knack for finding the best way through the forest when you're hiking together.

Talking About the Treasure

Talk about why this strength is valuable. For example, being a good listener makes people feel heard and understood, which is really important. It's like explaining why having a good sense of direction is super helpful in the woods—it can get you out of tricky situations and help everyone reach their destination safely.

Using the Gold

Encourage them to use their strengths in different parts of their life. If they're good at coming up with creative ideas, they might use this in solving a problem at work or planning a fun day out. It's like suggesting to someone good at navigating to take the lead in planning your hiking route.

Celebrating the Finds

Celebrate when they use their strengths. "You used your creativity to come up with a great solution—that's awesome!" It's like giving a high five when someone successfully leads the way on a hike, acknowledging their skill in action.

Adding More to the Collection

Encourage them to keep looking for and developing new strengths. Maybe they discover they're also good at making people laugh or organizing things. It's like finding new paths and treasures on each hike, adding to the adventure.

Continuing with the theme of recognizing and reinforcing client strengths, let's delve deeper into how this process can empower individuals and foster resilience and growth. Think of each person as a garden filled with various plants (strengths) that, when nurtured, can flourish and transform the landscape of their lives.

Cultivating a Growth Mindset

Encouraging a growth mindset is like preparing the soil for planting. It involves helping individuals understand that strengths can be developed with time and effort. You might say, "Just like a gardener cultivates their garden, you can cultivate your strengths. Every effort you make helps them grow stronger."

Identifying Hidden Strengths

Sometimes, strengths are hidden beneath the surface, like seeds waiting to sprout. Use discussions, activities, or reflections to help uncover these hidden gems. Ask questions like, "Can you think of a time you overcame a challenge? What abilities helped you through that?" This can reveal strengths they weren't aware of, much like discovering a seedling emerging from the ground.

Linking Strengths to Past Successes

Drawing connections between their strengths and past successes can reinforce their value. It's like showing someone how the fruits and flowers in their garden are the results of their careful tending to the plants. "Remember when you handled that difficult situation at work? Your problem-solving skills really shone through. That's a strength we can build on."

Strengths in Daily Life

Encourage applying these strengths in everyday scenarios, not just during big challenges. It's akin to using the herbs from your garden in daily cooking—it enhances the meal and reminds you of the garden's value. "How might your creativity in photography be applied to your current project at work? There might be an innovative approach just waiting to be discovered."

Creating a Strengths Portfolio

Help them create a "portfolio" of their strengths. This can be a list, a collage, or any creative form that represents their abilities. It's like keeping a garden journal where they note down the plants they have, their progress, and the beauty they bring. Reviewing this portfolio can boost confidence and remind them of their strengths during tough times.

Sharing Strengths with Others

Encourage sharing their strengths with others, whether through collaboration, teaching, or simply offering support. It's like sharing the bounty of your garden with neighbors. This not only reinforces the value of their strengths but also helps build community and connection.

Regular Reflection and Celebration

Set aside regular times to reflect on how they've used their strengths and to celebrate new growth. This could be through conversations, journaling, or any method that resonates with them. It's like taking a moment to appreciate the beauty of the garden you've cultivated, recognizing the new blooms, and planning for the next season.

Conclusion

Recognizing and reinforcing client strengths is about helping people see the valuable qualities they have inside, showing them why these qualities are important, and encouraging them to use these strengths in their daily lives. It's a way of building confidence and helping people navigate life's challenges with their own unique set of treasures.

Setting SMART goals in therapy.

Setting SMART goals in therapy is like planning a treasure hunt. You want to find the treasure, but to do that, you need a map that tells you exactly where to go, how to get there, what to look for, and when you plan to find it. SMART goals help you create that map. Let's break down what SMART stands for, using simple and easy-to-understand terms:

Specific

Your goal should be clear and specific, like saying, "I want to find the treasure chest under the big oak tree," instead of just, "I want to find treasure." In therapy, being specific might mean saying, "I want to feel more confident in social situations," rather than just, "I want to feel better."

Measurable

You need to know when you've found the treasure. Making your goal measurable means you can track your progress. It's like having clues along the way that show you're getting closer to the oak tree. In therapy, a measurable goal could be, "I want to start conversations with a new person at least once a week."

Achievable

Your treasure hunt should be something you can actually do. If the treasure is buried under a mountain, you need to have the right tools and skills to get there. Similarly, your goal should be realistic and attainable for you right now. For example, "I will join a social club this month to meet new people."

Relevant

The treasure hunt should matter to you; otherwise, why go on the adventure? Your goal should be relevant to your life and important to you. It's like choosing to search for a treasure that means something special, not just any old chest. A relevant goal in therapy might be, "Improving my social confidence will help me make new friends and feel less isolated."

Time-bound

Every good treasure hunt has a timeline. You decide, "I want to find the treasure by the end of summer." This keeps you focused and motivated. In therapy, setting a time-bound goal means saying, "I want to achieve this goal in the next three months." It gives you a clear deadline to work towards.

Putting It All Together

Let's say you're working on becoming more confident in social situations. A SMART goal could be: "I want to feel more confident talking to new people, so I will start one new conversation each week for the next two months during social club meetings."

Expanding on the concept of setting SMART goals in therapy, let's explore how this approach can be applied to various aspects of personal growth and overcoming challenges. Making your goals SMART is like equipping yourself with a compass, map, and a clear destination for your journey of self-improvement.

Breaking Down Complex Goals

Imagine you're facing a big, complex goal like "improve my mental health." That's like saying, "I want to explore the whole forest." It's a great ambition, but where do you start? By applying the SMART framework, you break this down into specific areas you want to improve, such as managing anxiety or improving sleep patterns. Each area becomes a path in the forest you plan to explore.

Specific Actions

For each path, decide on specific actions. If your goal is to manage anxiety, a specific action might be "practice deep breathing exercises for 10 minutes every morning." Just as a treasure map shows specific landmarks to look for, your actions should detail what you'll do to move toward your goal.

Tracking Progress

Measurable goals allow you to track your progress. It's like marking off the paths you've explored on your map. If your goal is to improve sleep, you might track how many hours you sleep each night or how often you follow your bedtime routine. Seeing progress, even small amounts, can be incredibly motivating.

Achieving Realistic Wins

Ensure your goals are achievable with the resources and skills you currently have. If you're juggling a busy schedule, a goal like "meditate for an hour every day" might not be realistic at first. Instead, starting with "meditate for 5 minutes each day" might be more doable, ensuring you feel successful and encouraged to continue.

Relevance to Your Life

Choose goals that are relevant and meaningful to you personally. If connecting with family is important to you, a goal might be "have a weekly dinner with family members." This ensures your efforts feel rewarding and directly contribute to your overall well-being and happiness.

Setting a Timeline

Adding a timeframe to your goals creates a sense of urgency and helps you prioritize. Saying "I will attend a social event at least once a month" gives you a clear timeframe to work within and helps prevent procrastination. It's like setting the date for when you plan to reach the treasure.

Adjusting as You Go

Remember, it's okay to adjust your goals as you progress. You might discover new paths in the forest you want to explore or realize some paths aren't as interesting as you thought. Revisiting and refining your goals ensures they remain aligned with what you truly want and need.

Why It Works

Using SMART goals in therapy is like having a detailed map for your treasure hunt. It guides you where you want to go, shows your progress, and keeps you motivated on your journey. Plus, it turns the vast and sometimes overwhelming goal of "feeling better" into smaller, achievable steps, making success not just a possibility but an expectation.

Conclusion

Setting SMART goals in therapy transforms the journey of personal growth into a structured adventure, with clear steps and milestones along the way. It turns the overwhelming into the achievable, guiding you through the forest of self-improvement with purpose and direction. By knowing exactly what you're aiming for, how you'll get there, and when you plan to arrive, you set yourself up for a rewarding journey that leads to real, meaningful change.

Example of Smart Goal during MI

Setting a SMART goal in Motivational Interviewing (MI) for helping a client named Alex who wants to reduce their alcohol consumption.

Specific

Goal: Alex wants to reduce their alcohol intake to improve their health and relationships.

Measurable

Criteria for Success: Alex decides to limit their drinking to no more than two drinks per occasion and to have at least four alcohol-free days each week.

Achievable

Action Plan: To achieve this goal, Alex will:

- Keep a diary to track their alcohol consumption daily.

- Identify triggers that lead to excessive drinking and develop alternative coping strategies, such as going for a walk or calling a friend.

- Attend a weekly support group meeting to connect with others who have similar goals.

Relevant

Why It Matters: Reducing alcohol intake is important to Alex because they've noticed negative effects on their health, including poor sleep and feeling lethargic. They also want to improve their relationships, which have been strained due to their drinking habits.

Time-bound

Deadline: Alex aims to achieve this new level of alcohol consumption within the next 3 months and will review their progress weekly to make any necessary adjustments.

Expanding on the example of helping Alex set a SMART goal in Motivational Interviewing (MI) to reduce their alcohol consumption, let's delve into how the therapist can support Alex throughout the process, ensuring the goal remains front and center in their journey toward change.

Regular Check-ins

Strategy: The therapist schedules regular check-ins with Alex to discuss progress, challenges, and any adjustments needed to the goal. This could be part of their weekly or bi-weekly sessions.

- **Application:** "Alex, let's take a few minutes to talk about how your goal went this week. What days were you successful in sticking to your limit, and what days were more challenging?"

Positive Reinforcement

Strategy: The therapist uses positive reinforcement to acknowledge Alex's efforts and successes, no matter how small, to build their motivation and confidence.

- **Application:** "I noticed you managed to stick to your goal during the weekend, which you mentioned was going to be challenging. That's a great achievement, and it shows your dedication to improving your health and relationships."

Reframing Setbacks

Strategy: When Alex encounters setbacks, the therapist helps reframe these as learning opportunities rather than failures, encouraging resilience and persistence.

- **Application:** "It sounds like Tuesday was a tough day, and you drank more than you intended. Let's explore what happened that day and how we can use this experience to strengthen your coping strategies."

Enhancing Coping Strategies

Strategy: The therapist works with Alex to develop and refine coping strategies for dealing with triggers and cravings, ensuring these strategies are practical and aligned with Alex's lifestyle.

- **Application:** "You mentioned that stress from work often leads you to drink. Let's brainstorm some stress-relief activities you can do instead of drinking, like exercise, meditation, or a hobby you enjoy."

Celebrating Milestones

Strategy: The therapist helps Alex set and celebrate milestones, breaking down the larger goal into smaller, achievable targets that provide a sense of progress.

- **Application:** "Reaching two weeks of sticking to your drinking goal is a milestone worth celebrating. How do you feel about your progress, and what can we do to acknowledge this achievement?"

Adjusting the Goal as Needed

Strategy: The therapist remains flexible, helping Alex adjust their goal if necessary, to ensure it continues to be realistic and relevant to their changing circumstances or insights.

- **Application:** "Now that you've had some time working toward your goal, do you feel it's still right for you, or are there adjustments we should consider to better suit your needs?"

Conclusion

Throughout the process, the therapist uses MI techniques to keep Alex engaged, motivated, and focused on their SMART goal. By maintaining an empathetic, supportive, and collaborative approach, the therapist helps Alex navigate the complexities of behavior change, making the journey toward reduced alcohol consumption a structured and empowering experience. This continuous support and adaptability are key to helping Alex achieve lasting change.

Case Study Simulation 1: Focusing a Scattered Conversation

Background: Chris is a 30-year-old software developer who sought therapy for anxiety and work-related stress. However, Chris often arrives at sessions overwhelmed and struggles to focus on a single issue, jumping from one topic to another. This scattering makes it challenging to address any one concern deeply.

Objective: Your goal as the therapist is to help Chris focus the conversation to effectively address and manage one concern at a time, improving their ability to cope with anxiety and stress.

Beginning of the Session

Therapist: "Chris, it's great to see you today. I've noticed that we often touch on many different topics during our sessions. While it's important to explore all that's on your mind, focusing on one main concern might help us make more progress. What's the most pressing issue for you right now?"

Chris: "I just feel swamped with everything. Work is crazy, my sleep is messed up, and I'm always worrying about the future. I don't even know where to start."

Establishing Focus

Therapist: "It sounds like you're dealing with a lot at once, which can definitely feel overwhelming. If we could pick one area to start with today, which one feels like it's impacting you the most?"

Chris: "Probably my work stress. It's like a domino effect on everything else."

Narrowing Down the Topic

Therapist: "Focusing on work stress is a good start. Can you tell me more about what specifically at work is causing you the most stress?"

Chris: "It's mainly the never-ending deadlines and feeling like I can't catch up. There's also this fear of not performing well enough."

Setting a Mini-Goal for the Session

Therapist: "Dealing with constant deadlines and fear of underperforming can be incredibly stressful. Let's set a mini-goal for today's session to explore strategies that might help you manage these pressures more effectively. How does that sound?"

Chris: "That sounds good. I really need some strategies."

Exploring and Refining Strategies

Therapist: "Let's break this down further. When you think about the deadlines, what's one small change you could make that might reduce your stress? For example, could setting more realistic deadlines with your team be an option?"

Chris: "Maybe I could talk to my manager about prioritizing tasks. I haven't really done that because I thought I needed to handle everything."

Encouraging Action and Reflection

Therapist: "Discussing task prioritization with your manager sounds like a positive step. How do you feel about trying that this week and observing how it impacts your stress levels?"

Chris: "I'm a bit nervous, but it's worth a try. I can't keep going like this."

Conclusion and Next Steps

Therapist: "Taking action, even if it's small, is a big step towards managing your work stress. Let's plan to discuss how the conversation with your manager goes in our next session. We can also explore other areas impacted by work stress, like your sleep, once we start seeing changes here. How does that plan sound to you?"

Chris: "It sounds like a plan. I feel a bit more hopeful having a specific action to take."

Summary

In this simulation, the therapist used techniques to focus a scattered conversation by identifying the most pressing issue, narrowing down the topic, setting a mini-goal for the session, exploring specific strategies, and planning next steps. This approach helped Chris feel more hopeful and empowered to take action, demonstrating the effectiveness of focusing on one concern at a time in therapy.

Case Study Simulation 2: Overcoming Procrastination and Time Management Issues

Background: Maya is a 25-year-old graduate student struggling with procrastination and time management, impacting her studies and increasing her stress levels. She often feels overwhelmed by her assignments and finds herself putting off work until the last minute, leading to panic and subpar submissions.

Objective: As Maya's therapist, your goal is to help her understand the root causes of her procrastination, develop better time management skills, and adopt strategies to keep her on track with her academic goals.

Beginning of the Session

Therapist: "Maya, it's good to see you today. You've mentioned feeling overwhelmed by your studies and struggling with procrastination. Can you tell me more about when you notice this happening the most?"

Maya: "It's usually when I have big assignments. I just can't seem to start them until it's almost too late. Then I'm rushing and stressed, and I know I'm not doing my best work."

Identifying Patterns

Therapist: "It sounds like larger tasks feel particularly daunting, leading you to delay starting them. Let's explore what thoughts or feelings come up for you when you think about beginning a big assignment."

Maya: "I guess I'm afraid I won't do it well, or it'll take forever. So, I just keep putting it off."

Setting a Focused Goal

Therapist: "That fear of not doing well or it taking too much time is common with procrastination. What if we worked on breaking down tasks into smaller, more manageable parts? This could help make starting less intimidating."

Maya: "That could help. I haven't really tried that; I always just see the whole thing and freeze."

Developing a Strategy

Therapist: "Let's create a plan for your next big assignment. We can break it down together and set mini-deadlines for each part. This way, you can focus on one small task at a time, making it more manageable. How does that sound?"

Maya: "That sounds doable. I'm willing to try it."

Implementing the Plan

Therapist: "Great. Let's start by outlining the assignment and identifying the first few steps. For each step, we'll set a specific, achievable goal and a mini-deadline. We'll also discuss what to do if you feel the urge to procrastinate."

Maya: "Okay, the first step could be just to draft an outline. I can do that in two days, maybe?"

Encouraging Reflection and Adjustment

Therapist: "Drafting an outline in two days is a great first step. Let's also plan a brief check-in, maybe through email, to see how you're feeling about the task and if the approach is working for you."

Maya: "That would be helpful. I think knowing I'll check in might keep me accountable."

Conclusion and Next Steps

Therapist: "We've set a clear, manageable plan for your next assignment. Remember, it's okay if everything doesn't go perfectly. The goal is to learn from the process and adjust as needed. How are you feeling about this approach?"

Maya: "I feel more optimistic. Having a plan and breaking it down actually makes it seem less scary."

Summary

In this case study, the therapist helped Maya address her procrastination and time management issues by understanding the underlying fears contributing to her behavior, setting a focused goal, and developing a step-by-step strategy with accountability measures. This approach aimed to make daunting tasks feel more manageable and to build Maya's confidence in her ability to manage her time and workload effectively.

Case Study Simulation 3: Enhancing Self-Esteem and Social Confidence

Background: Leo is a 32-year-old graphic designer who struggles with low self-esteem and social anxiety, which hinder his performance at work and his ability to form close relationships. Despite being talented, Leo often doubts his skills and avoids social situations for fear of judgment.

Objective: As Leo's therapist, your goal is to help him build self-esteem, enhance his social confidence, and develop strategies to manage anxiety in social settings.

Beginning of the Session

Therapist: "Leo, thank you for sharing your experiences with me. It sounds like these feelings of doubt and anxiety in social situations are really impacting your life. Let's explore what situations trigger these feelings the most. Can you give me an example?"

Leo: "Well, at work, whenever I have to present my designs, I just freeze up. I'm terrified of negative feedback. And outside of work, I avoid parties or gatherings because I'm scared I'll say something stupid."

Identifying Strengths

Therapist: "It's understandable how fear of judgment can be paralyzing. Let's also focus on your strengths. You mentioned your design work—what are some aspects of your job that you feel confident about?"

Leo: "I guess I'm really good at coming up with creative concepts. My colleagues often come to me for fresh ideas."

Setting a Focused Goal

Therapist: "Your creativity is a significant strength. How about we set a goal to build on this confidence at work and gradually apply it to social situations? For example, we could start by aiming for you to share one new idea in smaller group meetings without fearing the feedback."

Leo: "That sounds scary, but it might be good to start small like that."

Developing a Strategy

Therapist: "Let's break this down into steps. First, we could identify a safe opportunity for you to share your ideas, like in a one-on-one with a trusted colleague. What do you think?"

Leo: "I could probably try that with Maya; she's always been supportive."

Implementing the Plan

Therapist: "Perfect. Let's plan for you to share an idea with Maya this week. We'll also work on some strategies to manage the anxiety you might feel, like deep breathing exercises or positive self-talk before the meeting. How does that feel?"

Leo: "Nervous, but having a plan helps. I'm willing to try the exercises."

Encouraging Reflection and Adjustment

Therapist: "After you've had the meeting with Maya, let's reflect on how it went. We can discuss what felt challenging and what strategies helped. This will allow us to adjust our approach as needed. What are your thoughts on this?"

Leo: "I like the idea of reflecting afterward. It makes this feel more like a learning process."

Conclusion and Next Steps

Therapist: "Exactly, Leo. This is all about learning and growing at your own pace. By setting small, achievable goals and reflecting on your experiences, you'll gradually build confidence. Let's also consider joining a social skills group as a next step to practice in a supportive environment. How do you feel about that?"

Leo: "Joining a group sounds intimidating, but maybe it could be good for me. Let's talk more about it next time."

Summary

In this case study, the therapist helped Leo identify his strengths and set a focused, achievable goal to enhance his self-esteem and social confidence. By breaking down the goal into manageable steps and planning for reflection and adjustment, the therapist provided Leo with a structured approach to tackle his social anxiety, emphasizing growth and learning in a supportive, therapeutic environment.

Chapter 4: Evoking Client Motivation

Advanced techniques for eliciting change talk.

Eliciting change talk is a bit like being a coach who helps someone find their own reasons and motivation to change, rather than telling them what to do. Let's dive into some advanced techniques for bringing out change talk, all explained in a simple, friendly way.

1. Ask Evocative Questions

Imagine you're trying to help a friend figure out they want to start exercising more. Instead of asking, "Don't you think you should exercise more?" you could ask, "How would your life be different if you started exercising regularly?" This kind of question makes your friend think about the positive changes that could come from exercising, like feeling healthier or having more energy.

2. Use the Importance Ruler

This is like asking your friend, "On a scale of 1 to 10, how important is it for you to make this change?" If they say a number like 7, you can follow up with, "Why didn't you pick a lower number, like 4 or 5?" This makes your friend talk about what makes the change somewhat important to them, highlighting their own reasons for wanting to change.

3. Explore the Pros and Cons

It's like sitting down with your friend and drawing a big "T" on a piece of paper. On one side, you list the good things about changing (pros), and on the other, the not-so-good things about staying the same (cons). This helps your friend see the benefits of change and the drawbacks of not changing, encouraging them to talk more about why change might be good.

4. Look Back and Look Forward

This is like asking your friend to think about a time before they had this issue. You might say, "Can you remember a time when this wasn't a problem for you? What was different then?" Then, you ask them to imagine the future: "If you make this change, what do you hope will be different a year from now?" This gets your friend thinking about how much better things could be, which can motivate them to change.

5. Use Change Talk to Build More Change Talk

Whenever your friend says something that sounds like they want to change, like "I felt great when I went for a walk last week," use that as a stepping stone. You might say, "It sounds like that walk made you feel really good. What other activities could give you that feeling?" This encourages your friend to think more about positive changes and how to make them happen.

6. Summarize with a Twist

When you're summarizing what your friend has said, put a little spin on it that emphasizes their desire to change. If your friend mentioned feeling good after a walk and wanting to lose weight, you could say, "So, taking that walk made you feel great, and losing some weight is something you're looking to achieve for more of those good feelings." This reaffirms their reasons for change and encourages more discussion about it.

7. Reframe Negative Talk

Sometimes, people talk about what's going wrong without seeing the potential for change. Reframing is like taking a cloudy picture and adjusting the light to make it clearer and brighter. If your friend says, "I never have enough energy to get through my day," you might reframe it by saying, "It sounds like having more energy is really important to you. What do you think could help you feel more energized?" This shifts the focus from the problem to potential solutions.

8. The Miracle Question

This technique is like asking your friend to imagine a fairy tale where a magic wand makes everything better overnight. You ask, "If you woke up tomorrow and everything was exactly how you wanted it, what would be different?" This question helps them articulate their deepest desires for change, even if they haven't thought about them in concrete terms before.

9. Explore Values

People are more motivated to change when they see how it aligns with their deeper values. It's like choosing a path because you know it leads to a place you love. You might ask, "What's really important to you in life? How does making this change connect with those values?" This encourages them to see the change as a step towards living a life that's true to their core values.

10. Contrast Past Attempts

Discussing past attempts at change can reveal what motivates them and what barriers they face. It's like reviewing previous chapters of a book before deciding how the story should continue. "What have you tried before to make this change? What did you learn from those attempts?" This can help them identify what works, what doesn't, and how motivated they are to try a different approach.

11. Elicit Self-Motivational Statements

Encourage your friend to express in their own words why they want to change, how they might do it, and their belief in their ability to succeed. It's like encouraging them to tell their own story of change. "In what ways do you think making this change would benefit you? How confident are you that you can make this change?" Hearing themselves articulate these thoughts can strengthen their commitment to change.

12. Use Analogies and Metaphors

Sometimes, a well-chosen analogy or metaphor can help someone understand their situation and their potential for change more clearly. It's like using a story to illuminate a dark path. If your friend is struggling with fear of change, you might say, "Change can be like sailing to a new land. The journey might be rough, but think of the new worlds you could discover." This can help them visualize the process of change and its benefits in a more relatable way.

Conclusion

Advanced techniques for eliciting change talk are all about creativity, empathy, and strategic questioning. By helping someone explore their desires, fears, and values in depth, you empower them to articulate and embrace their own reasons for wanting to change. These methods don't just aim to start a conversation; they seek to spark a transformation, guiding the person to see the possibility of change as something that is not only desirable but achievable.

Overcoming resistance and sustaining talk.

Overcoming resistance and sustaining talk in Motivational Interviewing (MI) is like navigating a conversation with care and precision, ensuring you're both moving in the same direction without forcing the journey. MI emphasizes collaboration, respect for the client's autonomy, and drawing out the person's own motivations for change rather than imposing your own. Here are strategies to manage resistance and keep the conversation productive:

1. Express Empathy Through Reflective Listening

Empathy is the heart of MI. It involves genuinely trying to understand the world from the client's perspective and reflecting this understanding back to them. It's like saying, "I see the river you're navigating, and I'm here in the boat with you, not just watching from the shore." This approach helps reduce resistance because clients feel understood, not judged.

2. Develop Discrepancy

Clients may show resistance when they don't see a clear reason for change. Developing discrepancy involves helping them see the gap between where they are now and where they want to be. It's like gently pointing out that the current they're following might not lead to their desired destination. "You've mentioned wanting to lead a healthier lifestyle, yet it sounds like current habits might be steering you away from that goal. What are your thoughts on this?"

3. Roll with Resistance

Instead of confronting resistance directly, MI teaches us to roll with it. When you encounter resistance, don't push against it. Instead, use it as a cue to change direction in the conversation or delve deeper into understanding the client's perspective. It's akin to paddling gently along with the current to find a smoother path rather than fighting against the waves. "It seems like this topic is a bit uncomfortable. Would you like to explore what makes it feel that way, or should we shift our focus for now?"

4. Support Self-efficacy

Belief in one's ability to change is crucial. Encouraging and supporting self-efficacy in clients helps them overcome resistance by building confidence. It's like reminding someone who's hesitant to navigate the rapids that they've successfully navigated similar challenges before. "You've shown a lot of strength in dealing with challenges in the past. How can we harness that strength as you think about making this change?"

5. Affirmations

Positive reinforcement can motivate clients to continue engaging in change talk. Highlighting a client's strengths and past successes reinforces their capability to change. It's like acknowledging every successful maneuver through the rapids, reinforcing their skill and courage. "I'm impressed by your willingness to examine this issue so openly. It shows a lot of courage and insight."

6. Summarize and Guide

Periodically summarizing the conversation helps clarify the client's motivations and the discussion's direction. It also provides an opportunity to gently steer back towards change talk if the conversation has veered off course. Think of it as periodically checking the map together to ensure you're still on the path to treasure. "Let me make sure I've got this right... You're saying that while change is daunting, there's also a part of you that's eager for a different lifestyle. Is that correct?"

7. Ask Permission Before Offering Advice

In MI, advice is offered gently and usually only after seeking the client's permission. This respects the client's autonomy and reduces resistance because they're open to hearing your perspective. It's like asking, "There's a side path here that might be worth exploring. Would you like to check it out?"

Conclusion

In MI, overcoming resistance and sustaining talk is about moving in harmony with the client, using empathy, strategic questioning, and affirmation to navigate the conversation toward change. It's a collaborative journey where the client's autonomy is respected, and their own motivations for change are brought to the forefront, making the journey toward change a shared adventure.

Hope and confidence in evoking motivation.

In Motivational Interviewing (MI), hope and confidence are pivotal in sparking the desire for change and fueling the journey towards achieving it. They are especially crucial because MI focuses on eliciting and strengthening a person's own motivation for change, rather than imposing external motivations.

The Role of Hope in MI

Hope in MI acts as the beacon that lights the way forward. It's the belief that change is possible and that a better future can be achieved. Without hope, the idea of change can seem daunting or pointless.

Example in MI: Consider Jamie, who is struggling with substance abuse and feels trapped in a cycle of attempts and failures to quit. During an MI session, the therapist listens empathetically and shares stories of others who have successfully overcome similar challenges, carefully avoiding creating any pressure to change. This approach helps Jamie to see that change is indeed possible, igniting a spark of hope. The therapist might say, "Many people who've felt stuck as you do now have found their path to a healthier life. What do you think could be different for you if things were to change?"

The Role of Confidence in MI

Confidence in MI is about building the individual's belief in their own ability to make these changes. It's grounded in the person's past successes and strengths, reinforcing the idea that they have the power to alter their course.

Example in MI: Continuing with Jamie's story, the therapist helps Jamie identify past successes, even those not related to substance use, and explores how the skills and strengths from those successes could be applied to their current situation. For example, the therapist might highlight Jamie's perseverance in completing a challenging work project or their commitment to being a supportive friend. "You've shown you can set your mind to difficult tasks and see them through. How might those strengths support you in making the changes you're considering now?"

Hope and Confidence Together in MI

When hope and confidence are woven together in MI, they create a powerful combination that can significantly boost motivation. Hope shows the individual that a different future is possible, while confidence reassures them that they have the means to reach it.

Integrated Example in MI: In subsequent sessions, Jamie begins to articulate personal reasons for wanting to change, drawing on the hope that change is possible and the growing confidence in their own abilities. They might start setting small, achievable goals, with the therapist using MI techniques to reinforce Jamie's belief in their ability to achieve these goals. "Given your determination and the steps you've already taken, how do you feel about your ability to continue making changes?"

Conclusion

In MI, fostering hope and confidence is not about guaranteeing success or denying the realities of the challenges ahead. It's about helping individuals see that change is possible (hope) and that they have the strengths and abilities required to pursue it (confidence). This approach supports the core MI principle that motivation for change is most potent when it comes from within the individual, making hope and confidence critical elements in the motivational process.

Case Study Simulation 1: Motivating a demoralized client.

Background: Ella is a 40-year-old who has been struggling with job dissatisfaction and a recent breakup. These challenges have left her feeling demoralized and unsure about her future. She has started to question her worth and her ability to make positive changes in her life.

Objective: As Ella's therapist using Motivational Interviewing (MI), your goal is to help Ella find her internal motivation to overcome her current state of demoralization, focusing on rebuilding her self-esteem and envisioning a hopeful future.

Beginning of the Session

Therapist: "Ella, I appreciate you opening up about how you're feeling. It sounds like you're going through a really tough time with your job and personal life. It's understandable to feel demoralized when facing such challenges. What's one thing that you wish were different right now?"

Ella: "I just wish I could feel happy again. I don't see how that's possible with everything going wrong."

Expressing Empathy and Understanding

Therapist: "It's tough to envision feeling happy when you're in the midst of so much. It's okay to feel this way, and it's also okay to take small steps toward where you want to be. Has there ever been a time in the past when you've felt similarly stuck but found a way through it?"

Ella: "Well, yes, a few years back, I felt stuck in my career but then I took some courses and that really helped. I just don't have the energy for that now."

Building on Past Successes

Therapist: "It's great that you were able to find a way through a tough time before. It shows you have resilience and the capacity to make changes that matter to you. Even though it feels different now, you still have those strengths. What small step could feel manageable to you right now, something that might help you start to feel a bit better?"

Ella: "Maybe I could start reading again. I used to love that."

Fostering Hope and Confidence

Therapist: "Reading sounds like a wonderful place to start. It can be a source of comfort and a step toward reclaiming something you love. How do you think incorporating reading into your routine could impact your current feelings?"

Ella: "It might help me relax a bit more, take my mind off things."

Setting a Specific Goal

Therapist: "That's a good insight. Setting aside time to read each day can be a simple, yet effective way to start changing how you feel. How much time do you think you could comfortably set aside for reading each day?"

Ella: "I think I could manage 30 minutes before bed."

Supporting Self-Efficacy

Therapist: "Thirty minutes sounds perfect. It's a manageable goal that can have a positive impact on your day. I believe in your ability to make this change. How do you feel about this plan?"

Ella: "It feels doable, maybe even something to look forward to."

Conclusion and Next Steps

Therapist: "Having something to look forward to can be a powerful motivator. Let's check in on this next time we meet. We can also explore other activities or changes you might want to consider, always at your pace. Remember, each small step is progress."

Summary

In this simulation, the therapist used MI techniques to connect with Ella, focusing on understanding her feelings of demoralization, reminding her of past successes to build confidence, and helping her set a realistic and specific goal to reintroduce happiness into her life gradually. This approach aims to motivate Ella by fostering hope, enhancing her self-efficacy, and gently guiding her towards envisioning and working towards a more positive future.

Case Study Simulation 2: Building Resilience in Facing Career Challenges

Background: Jordan is a 35-year-old marketing professional who has recently been passed over for a promotion they felt they deserved. This setback has significantly impacted Jordan's confidence and motivation at work, leading to feelings of inadequacy and thoughts of giving up on their career aspirations.

Objective: As Jordan's therapist using Motivational Interviewing (MI), your goal is to help Jordan rebuild their confidence, rediscover their motivation, and develop resilience in the face of career setbacks.

Beginning of the Session

Therapist: "Jordan, thank you for sharing your experiences with me. It sounds like not getting the promotion has been really tough on you, shaking your confidence in your abilities and future prospects. What was your initial reaction when you heard the news?"

Jordan: "I was devastated. I've put everything into my job, and it felt like it was all for nothing. I've started questioning if I'm even in the right career."

Expressing Empathy and Exploring Impact

Therapist: "Feeling devastated in such a situation is completely understandable. It sounds like this has not only affected your view of your job but also your perception of your career path. When these doubts come up, what are some thoughts that go through your mind?"

Jordan: "I wonder if all my hard work is even recognized or worth it. Maybe I'm not as good as I thought I was."

Reframing and Recognizing Strengths

Therapist: "It's natural to question your worth after such a disappointment, yet the dedication and hard work you've shown are significant strengths. Can you think of a time when your effort was recognized, or you felt particularly proud of your work?"

Jordan: "Well, there was a campaign last year that was almost canceled, but I managed to turn it around, and it ended up being one of the most successful ones we've had."

Building on Past Successes

Therapist: "That's a fantastic achievement and a testament to your skills and dedication. Let's use that experience as a foundation. What strengths did you draw on to make that campaign successful?"

Jordan: "Creativity, persistence, and I guess, leadership. I had to convince my team to stick with it and see it through."

Fostering Hope and Setting Goals

Therapist: "Those are valuable strengths not just for your current role but for any career aspirations you have. Holding onto that creativity, persistence, and leadership, what's one small step you can take this week to start rebuilding your confidence at work?"

Jordan: "Maybe I could propose a new project, something I've been thinking about but haven't acted on yet."

Supporting Self-Efficacy

Therapist: "Proposing a new project sounds like an excellent way to reengage and showcase your strengths. How confident do you feel about putting this idea forward, and what support might you need to do it?"

Jordan: "I'm a bit nervous, but discussing the campaign I turned around has reminded me that I can do this. Maybe I could use some help refining my proposal."

Conclusion and Next Steps

Therapist: "Let's focus on preparing that proposal then. Remember, your value doesn't diminish because of one setback. You have a track record of success to build on. How about we look at refining your proposal together next session?"

Summary

In this case study, the therapist used MI to help Jordan navigate through their feelings of defeat and self-doubt following a career setback. By empathetically exploring Jordan's reactions, highlighting past successes, and identifying inherent strengths, the therapist helped Jordan begin to rebuild confidence. Setting a tangible goal of proposing a new project provided a concrete step for Jordan to take action, fostering a sense of hope and self-efficacy essential for overcoming challenges and building resilience.

Case Study Simulation 3: Enhancing Social Skills and Reducing Anxiety

Background: Sara is a 28-year-old software engineer who struggles with social anxiety, which affects her performance in team meetings and her ability to form connections with colleagues. Despite being highly skilled in her job, Sara feels isolated at work and worries this might hinder her career progression.

Objective: As Sara's therapist using Motivational Interviewing (MI), your goal is to help Sara develop strategies to manage her social anxiety, enhance her social skills, and build confidence in her interactions at work.

Beginning of the Session

Therapist: "Sara, it's great to see you today. You've mentioned feeling anxious in social situations at work, which seems to be impacting your sense of connection with colleagues. Can you tell me about a recent situation where you felt this anxiety?"

Sara: "In our last team meeting, I had some ideas I thought could really help our project, but I just couldn't bring myself to speak up. I kept worrying about saying something wrong."

Expressing Empathy and Validating Feelings

Therapist: "That sounds like a challenging situation, feeling like you have valuable contributions but being held back by these worries. It's understandable to feel anxious about how others might perceive you, especially in a professional setting. How does this anxiety typically affect you in those moments?"

Sara: "My heart races, and I get so caught up in my worries that I end up not saying anything at all. It's frustrating."

Exploring Ambivalence

Therapist: "It sounds like there's a part of you that really wants to engage and contribute, but the anxiety creates a barrier. If you felt more confident in these situations, what would be different for you?"

Sara: "I'd be able to share my ideas, contribute more to the team, and maybe even feel more connected with my colleagues."

Building on Strengths

Therapist: "You've already shown a lot of courage by recognizing this challenge and seeking to address it. Reflecting on times you have successfully engaged with others, even in small ways, what strengths did you draw on in those situations?"

Sara: "I guess I'm pretty good at listening and providing thoughtful feedback when others ask for it directly."

Setting a Focused Goal

Therapist: "Using those strengths as a starting point, let's think about a small, achievable goal for the next team meeting. Perhaps you could plan to share one piece of feedback or one idea, using your listening skills as a foundation. How does that sound?"

Sara: "That seems less daunting. I could probably manage that."

Developing a Strategy

Therapist: "Let's brainstorm some strategies to help manage the anxiety you feel in the moment. For example, some people find it helpful to practice deep breathing exercises or to prepare their points in advance. What approach do you think might work best for you?"

Sara: "Preparing my points in advance could help. It might make me feel more confident about what I'm going to say."

Conclusion and Next Steps

Therapist: "Preparing in advance is a great strategy. Let's also think about a small reward for yourself after sharing your ideas, something to look forward to. We can review how it went in our next session and explore further steps to build on this progress. Remember, each small step is a victory."

Summary

In this case study, the therapist used MI to help Sara address her social anxiety and its impact on her workplace interactions. By empathizing with her experiences, validating her feelings, and helping her identify her own strengths, the therapist supported Sara in setting a realistic goal for enhancing her social participation. Developing a specific strategy for achieving this goal provided Sara with a clear path forward, empowering her to take actionable steps toward overcoming her anxiety and improving her social skills in a professional setting.

Chapter 5: Planning for Change

Collaboratively developing a plan for change.

In Motivational Interviewing (MI), collaboratively developing a plan for change is akin to joining hands with someone to map out a journey they've decided to embark on. This process emphasizes partnership, respect, and the client's autonomy, ensuring the plan aligns with their values, strengths, and readiness for change. Here's how this collaborative process unfolds:

1. Setting the Destination Together

First, it's crucial to clarify the goal or change the client wishes to achieve. This is done through a process of exploration and discussion, ensuring the goal is specific, meaningful, and resonates with the client's personal values.

- **Example:** If a client wants to improve their physical health, you'd work together to define what this means for them. Does it involve losing weight, eating healthier, exercising more, or a combination of these?

2. Mapping the Route

Once the destination is clear, the next step is to map out the route. This involves brainstorming different paths to the goal, evaluating each for its feasibility, and considering the client's preferences and life circumstances.

- **Example:** For achieving better physical health, you might explore various options like joining a gym, finding a workout buddy, planning healthier meals, or setting a step count goal with a pedometer.

3. Identifying Milestones

Milestones are like checkpoints along the journey that help the client see progress. These should be smaller, achievable goals that lead up to the main goal, providing motivation and a sense of accomplishment along the way.

- **Example:** If the ultimate goal is to lose 20 pounds, milestones might include losing the first 5 pounds, consistently exercising three times a week for a month, or successfully avoiding sugary snacks for two weeks.

4. Equipping for the Journey

This step involves identifying skills, resources, and strategies the client will need to navigate the path to change. It's about ensuring they have the right tools in their backpack.

- **Example:** To support a goal of healthier eating, you might discuss meal planning strategies, identify healthy recipes, or explore ways to manage cravings.

5. Planning for Obstacles

Anticipating and planning for potential obstacles is crucial. Discuss what might derail the journey and strategize on how to navigate these challenges or adjust the plan as needed.

- **Example:** If time management is a potential barrier to exercising, you could explore ways to integrate activity into the client's daily routine or identify shorter, more intense workouts.

6. Reviewing and Adjusting the Plan

A key principle of MI is flexibility. The plan should be reviewed regularly, celebrating successes, learning from setbacks, and making adjustments based on the client's experiences and feedback.

- **Example:** If the client finds certain dietary changes too restrictive, you might work together to find a more balanced approach that still aligns with their health goals.

7. Reinforcing Autonomy and Support

Throughout this process, it's important to reinforce the client's autonomy by emphasizing that they are in control of their choices and actions. Providing unwavering support and encouragement helps bolster their confidence and commitment to change.

- **Example:** Reminding the client that they have the freedom to choose how they meet their physical health goals and acknowledging their efforts and progress reinforces their autonomy and motivation.

Conclusion

Collaboratively developing a plan for change in MI is about building a personalized roadmap that guides the client from where they are to where they want to be. By working together to set the destination, map the route, prepare for the journey, and navigate challenges, you help the client move towards their goal with confidence, motivation, and a sense of ownership over their change process.

Integrating MI with treatment planning

Integrating Motivational Interviewing (MI) with treatment planning and intervention is like blending the art of engaging and motivating clients with the science of structured treatment approaches. It's about using the empathetic, client-centered communication style of MI to enhance the effectiveness of more structured treatment plans. Here's how this integration can work, explained in a straightforward, easy-to-understand manner:

1. Establishing Rapport and Exploring Ambivalence

Before diving into a specific treatment plan, use MI techniques to build a strong therapeutic alliance and explore any ambivalence the client may have about change. This initial step ensures that the client feels heard and understood, setting a positive tone for the collaboration.

- **Example:** In a substance abuse treatment plan, before outlining the steps of the intervention, spend time discussing the client's mixed feelings about reducing substance use, emphasizing their autonomy and understanding their perspective.

2. Setting Collaborative Goals

Incorporate MI by collaboratively setting treatment goals with the client. This means working together to identify goals that are meaningful and motivating to the client, rather than imposing predetermined goals on them.

- **Example:** For a client dealing with anxiety, rather than prescribing a set of activities, ask what aspects of their life they would most like to improve. Use their input to shape the goals of cognitive-behavioral therapy (CBT) interventions, such as tackling specific fears or social situations.

3. Eliciting Change Talk

Throughout the treatment process, use MI strategies to elicit and reinforce change talk. This involves guiding conversations in a way that encourages the client to express their desires, abilities, reasons, and need for change, reinforcing their motivation.

- **Example:** In a weight loss program, regularly invite the client to discuss their reasons for wanting to lose weight, their vision of a healthier lifestyle, and the steps they feel capable of taking, aligning these with the dietary and exercise plans.

4. Strengthening Commitment

Use MI to strengthen the client's commitment to the treatment plan. This can be done by summarizing their expressed motivations and plans, asking for commitment, and exploring what might help them stay committed.

- **Example:** In managing depression, after agreeing on a plan that includes medication, therapy, and lifestyle changes, revisit the client's reasons for wanting to feel better and ask how committed they feel to their plan, discussing ways to overcome potential barriers.

5. Integrating Client Feedback

Make the treatment plan dynamic by regularly integrating client feedback, an approach consistent with MI. Adjust the plan based on the client's experiences, successes, and challenges, maintaining an open dialogue about what's working and what isn't.

- **Example:** If a client is struggling with adherence to a medication regimen, discuss their concerns and experiences openly, and collaboratively explore adjustments, whether in timing, reminders, or understanding the medication's role in their broader health goals.

6. Planning for Setbacks

Anticipate and plan for setbacks within the treatment plan, using MI to discuss how these will be addressed. This preparation helps maintain motivation and commitment by framing setbacks as opportunities for learning and growth.

- **Example:** In addiction recovery, proactively discuss potential relapse scenarios, emphasizing that a relapse isn't a failure but a step in the learning process. Together, develop a plan for addressing and learning from setbacks.

7. Reinforcing Progress

Consistently acknowledge and reinforce progress towards treatment goals, using MI to highlight the client's strengths and successes. This positive reinforcement helps build confidence and sustains motivation.

- **Example:** In a program for managing chronic pain, regularly highlight the client's efforts and achievements in using coping strategies, physical therapy exercises, or medication management, linking these successes back to their personal goals and motivations.

Conclusion

Integrating MI with treatment planning and intervention transforms the treatment process into a more personalized, dynamic, and collaborative journey. It leverages the client's own motivation and strengths to foster engagement and commitment to their goals, enhancing the effectiveness of structured treatment approaches through empathy, respect, and partnership.

Anticipating challenges and planning for setbacks.

Anticipating challenges and planning for setbacks in the context of behavior change or therapy is like preparing for a hike through unpredictable terrain. Just as a hiker packs extra supplies and maps out alternative routes in advance, individuals working towards change can prepare for potential obstacles and plan how to navigate them. This preparation is crucial for maintaining progress and resilience. Here's how to approach this process in simple terms:

1. Identify Potential Challenges

Start by brainstorming possible challenges or setbacks that could occur during the journey of change. It's like checking the weather and trail conditions before a hike. For someone trying to quit smoking, challenges might include high-stress situations, social events with other smokers, or moments of strong cravings.

2. Develop Strategies for Each Challenge

For each identified challenge, develop specific strategies or actions to overcome or manage it. This is akin to packing rain gear for bad weather or bringing a compass for navigation. If stress is a trigger for smoking, strategies might include practicing mindfulness, having a list of stress-relief activities ready, or using a stress ball.

3. Create a Support Plan

Determine what kind of support will be helpful and how to access it when challenges arise. This could involve identifying supportive friends or family members, joining a support group, or knowing how to reach out to a therapist or counselor. It's like having an emergency contact list or joining a hiker's group for mutual support.

4. Set Realistic Expectations

Understand that setbacks are a natural part of the change process, not failures. Adjusting expectations is like acknowledging that some parts of the hike will be tough, and it's okay to rest or take a slower pace. This mindset helps maintain motivation and self-compassion when faced with difficulties.

5. Practice Coping Skills

Before facing a challenge, practice the coping skills and strategies that have been identified. This is similar to training or doing smaller hikes to prepare for a big one. Practicing deep breathing, role-playing difficult situations, or rehearsing positive self-talk can build confidence and effectiveness in using these skills.

6. Plan for Quick Recovery

Create a plan for how to get back on track quickly after a setback. This might include steps to reflect on what happened, learn from the experience, and recommit to the goals. It's like knowing the nearest exit points or rest areas along a hike, allowing for a safe and swift return to the path.

7. Celebrate Progress

Recognize and celebrate progress, not just the absence of setbacks. Celebrating milestones, no matter how small, reinforces the value of the effort being made. It's like taking a moment to enjoy the view or celebrate reaching a checkpoint, acknowledging the hard work and progress made.

Let's consider the example of Maya, who is working on managing her anxiety, a common goal that many people share. Maya has decided to use techniques like mindfulness meditation, regular exercise, and seeking support from friends when she's feeling overwhelmed. Here's how she anticipates challenges and plans for setbacks in her journey:

Identifying Potential Challenges

Maya knows that work deadlines and social gatherings are significant triggers for her anxiety. She also recognizes that skipping her exercise routine or meditation sessions can increase her anxiety levels.

Developing Strategies for Each Challenge

For work deadlines, Maya decides to break down projects into smaller tasks and set realistic timelines for each, reducing the overwhelm. For social gatherings, she plans to set boundaries for how long she stays and practices grounding techniques before attending to help manage her anxiety.

Creating a Support Plan

Maya identifies a close friend who understands her anxiety issues and agrees to be her go-to person when she needs to talk. She also joins an online support group for people dealing with anxiety to share experiences and coping strategies.

Setting Realistic Expectations

Maya acknowledges that her anxiety won't disappear overnight and that some days will be harder than others. She accepts that there might be setbacks but views them as part of her learning and growth process.

Practicing Coping Skills

Before attending a social event, Maya practices deep breathing exercises and visualizes a positive experience to reduce her anticipatory anxiety. She also schedules short, daily mindfulness sessions to build her skill in managing anxious thoughts.

Plan for Quick Recovery

Maya decides that if she has a particularly anxious day or if she misses her exercise or meditation, she won't berate herself. Instead, she'll focus on understanding what happened and how she can adjust her plan moving forward. She commits to resuming her routine the next day without dwelling on the setback.

Celebrate Progress

Maya keeps a journal where she records her successes, no matter how small. Whether it's managing to stay at a social event for her intended time, completing a work project without undue stress, or just sticking to her meditation routine for a week straight, she acknowledges and celebrates these wins.

Conclusion

In this example, Maya's approach to managing her anxiety incorporates anticipating challenges and planning for setbacks. By identifying her triggers, developing specific strategies, creating a support network, setting realistic expectations, practicing coping skills, planning for recovery from setbacks, and celebrating her progress, Maya is well-equipped to navigate her journey toward better managing her anxiety. This holistic and proactive approach enhances her resilience and maintains her motivation, even when she encounters obstacles.

Anticipating challenges and planning for setbacks equips individuals with the tools and mindset needed to navigate the complex journey of change. It acknowledges that the path won't always be smooth, but with preparation and support, obstacles can be overcome, and progress can continue. This approach fosters resilience, encouraging individuals to keep moving forward, even when the terrain gets tough.

Case Study Simulation 1: Crafting a change plan with a reluctant client.

Background: Alex is a 45-year-old who has been referred to therapy by their primary care doctor due to concerns about high blood pressure and stress management. Alex acknowledges the need for lifestyle changes but expresses reluctance, citing a demanding job, family responsibilities, and little free time as major barriers to change.

Objective: As Alex's therapist using Motivational Interviewing (MI), your goal is to collaboratively craft a change plan that addresses these concerns, focusing on manageable and realistic steps that Alex feels capable of taking.

Beginning of the Session

Therapist: "Alex, thank you for sharing your concerns with me today. It sounds like you're facing some real challenges in finding time for yourself amidst your job and family duties. Given your doctor's concerns, how do you feel about making some changes to manage your stress and improve your health?"

Alex: "I know I need to do something, but I honestly don't see how I can fit anything else into my schedule. It feels impossible."

Expressing Empathy and Exploring Ambivalence

Therapist: "It sounds like you're feeling stuck between knowing changes are needed and feeling overwhelmed by your current commitments. That must be really tough. If there were a way to make small changes without disrupting your schedule too much, what would you think about that?"

Alex: "I'd be open to it, but it has to be really manageable. I can't commit to anything big right now."

Identifying Strengths and Past Successes

Therapist: "Let's focus on your strengths and any small steps you've successfully integrated into your life before, no matter how minor they might seem. Can you recall any changes you've made in the past that you found beneficial?"

Alex: "Well, I started taking the stairs at work a few months back instead of the elevator. That's something, I guess."

Setting a Focused Goal

Therapist: "Taking the stairs is a great example of a small but impactful change. Building on that, can you think of another small adjustment you might be willing to try, perhaps related to managing stress or your health more broadly?"

Alex: "Maybe I could try some of those breathing exercises for stress. I've read they don't take much time."

Developing a Strategy

Therapist: "Breathing exercises are an excellent choice. They can be done almost anywhere, anytime, and they're effective for stress reduction. How about we start with just three minutes a day? We can identify a specific time that works for you to integrate this into your routine."

Alex: "I could do that first thing in the morning, before the day gets away from me."

Planning for Obstacles

Therapist: "Morning sounds like a good plan. Let's also think about what might make it hard to stick to this routine and how you can address these challenges. For example, what if you have an unusually early meeting?"

Alex: "I guess I could do the breathing exercises after the meeting or even during my commute."

Conclusion and Next Steps

Therapist: "That's a flexible approach, adapting to the day's needs. Let's check in on how this is going in our next session. We can discuss what's working, what isn't, and adjust as needed. How does that sound?"

Alex: "Sounds good. I think I can manage that."

Summary

In this case study, the therapist used MI to help Alex move from a place of reluctance to being open to making a small, manageable change. By expressing empathy, identifying a specific and achievable goal, planning for potential obstacles, and agreeing on a simple strategy, the therapist supported Alex in taking a first step towards better health and stress management. This approach emphasizes the importance of client autonomy and the power of small changes, setting the foundation for further progress in future sessions.

Case Study Simulation 2: Addressing Sleep Difficulties

Background: Jordan is a 38-year-old graphic designer who has been experiencing difficulties falling asleep and staying asleep for several months. This sleep issue has started to affect Jordan's productivity at work and overall mood. Jordan is aware of the problem but feels overwhelmed by the thought of making changes to improve sleep, partly due to a belief that work demands make it impossible to have a healthier bedtime routine.

Objective: As Jordan's therapist using Motivational Interviewing (MI), your goal is to help Jordan recognize the importance of addressing sleep issues, identify manageable steps to improve sleep hygiene, and build confidence in their ability to implement these changes.

Beginning of the Session

Therapist: "Jordan, I appreciate you bringing up your sleep challenges today. It sounds like this has been a tough area for you, impacting many aspects of your life. What are your thoughts on how your sleep affects your daily routine?"

Jordan: "It's been rough. I know I should be getting more sleep, but I just keep staying up late with work, and then when I try to sleep, I can't switch off."

Expressing Empathy and Exploring Ambivalence

Therapist: "That sounds incredibly frustrating, feeling caught in this cycle of wanting to rest but feeling compelled to keep working late. It's like your mind keeps racing even when you know it's time to wind down. What would it mean for you to break this cycle?"

Jordan: "It'd be a game-changer. I'd probably be less cranky, more focused, and just... happier, I guess. But it feels impossible right now."

Identifying Values and Discrepancies

Therapist: "Being less cranky, more focused, and happier sounds like important goals for you. It seems there's a gap between where you are now and where you'd like to be in terms of your well-being. Reflecting on this, what small changes do you think could help bridge this gap?"

Jordan: "Maybe I could start by actually shutting down my computer and not working from bed. I've heard that helps."

Setting a Focused Goal

Therapist: "That's a solid first step, creating a clear boundary between work and rest. How do you feel about implementing this change over the next week?"

Jordan: "I think I can do that. It's going to be hard, but I'm willing to try."

Developing a Strategy

Therapist: "Let's think about a strategy to make this more manageable. Perhaps you could set an alarm as a reminder to turn off your computer at a specific time each evening. What time do you think would be realistic for you to end your workday?"

Jordan: "Maybe 9 PM? That gives me an hour to wind down before I try to sleep at 10."

Therapist: "9 PM sounds like a practical goal. Setting an alarm as a cue to begin your wind-down routine can help signal to your brain that it's time to transition from work mode to rest mode. How do you feel about also creating a relaxing pre-sleep routine to help you wind down?"

Jordan: "I like that idea. Maybe I could read something light or do some gentle stretching instead of scrolling through my phone."

Therapist: "Incorporating relaxing activities like reading or stretching sounds perfect for signaling to your body it's time to rest. Let's also discuss what you might do if you find yourself wanting to work past 9 PM. How can you remind yourself of the importance of sticking to your new routine?"

Jordan: "I could keep a note by my computer reminding me why I'm doing this – to be less irritable, more focused at work, and overall happier."

Therapist: "That's a great strategy, using a visual reminder of your goals to help stay on track. It's also important to be kind to yourself if there are nights when things don't go as planned. Reflecting on any slip-ups can be valuable, helping us understand what might work better next time. How do you feel about this approach?"

Jordan: "It makes me feel more hopeful. Knowing that it's okay to have off nights takes off some pressure."

Therapist: "Absolutely, progress isn't linear, and self-compassion is key. Next session, we can review how the week went, what worked well, and what challenges you encountered. We'll adjust the plan as needed based on your experience. How does that sound for a starting point?"

Jordan: "It sounds good. I'm actually looking forward to trying this out and seeing if it makes a difference."

Therapist: "I'm glad to hear that, Jordan. Remember, this is about making small, sustainable changes that lead to significant improvements in your well-being. I'm here to support you through this process."

Summary

In this case study, the therapist uses MI to help Jordan navigate their sleep difficulties by expressing empathy, exploring ambivalence, and collaboratively setting a focused, achievable goal. By developing a practical strategy for implementing this change and planning for potential setbacks, the therapist supports Jordan in taking the first steps toward improved sleep hygiene. This approach emphasizes the importance of flexibility, self-compassion, and gradual progress in facilitating sustainable behavior change.

Chapter 6: Mastering Complex Conversations

Navigating dual diagnoses and comorbidities

Navigating dual diagnoses and comorbidities in Motivational Interviewing (MI) requires a nuanced, empathetic approach that recognizes the complexities of managing multiple health issues simultaneously. It's akin to juggling: the therapist and client work together to keep all balls in the air, understanding that the way one issue is handled can affect the others. Here's a simplified explanation of how MI can be applied in such complex scenarios:

Understanding the Interconnectedness

First, it's crucial to understand how the diagnoses interact with each other. For instance, depression can exacerbate substance abuse, and vice versa. In MI, the therapist helps the client explore these connections, fostering an understanding of how addressing one issue may positively impact the others.

- **Example:** If a client has anxiety and a smoking addiction, the therapist might explore how anxiety triggers the need to smoke and discuss how reducing smoking might initially increase anxiety levels, planning strategies to manage this.

Prioritizing Issues

With multiple issues at play, it's important to collaboratively identify which issue(s) the client feels most ready to tackle. This doesn't mean ignoring the other diagnoses but rather choosing a starting point that will build momentum and confidence.

- **Example:** A client struggling with obesity and depression may decide to focus on physical activity as a starting point, which can have mood-lifting benefits and contribute to weight management, addressing both concerns simultaneously.

Setting Realistic, Integrated Goals

Goals should reflect the reality of dealing with multiple diagnoses. They should be flexible, achievable, and integrated to address the complexity of the client's situation.

- **Example:** For someone managing diabetes and experiencing major depressive disorder, goals might include a manageable exercise routine that fits their energy levels and dietary changes that consider both blood sugar management and mood stabilization.

Tailoring MI Techniques

Using MI techniques, such as reflective listening and eliciting change talk, should be tailored to acknowledge the challenges and motivations related to each diagnosis. This can help in building a holistic change plan that the client is genuinely motivated to follow.

- **Example:** Reflective listening can be used to validate the difficulties of adhering to a medication regimen for bipolar disorder while managing the impulsivity of a co-occurring substance use disorder, gently guiding the conversation towards strategies for improvement.

Developing Coping Strategies

Identify and develop coping strategies that can be applied across diagnoses, enhancing resilience and self-efficacy. This might involve stress reduction techniques, improving social support networks, or cognitive-behavioral strategies to manage negative thought patterns.

- **Example:** Teaching mindfulness techniques can help a client with chronic pain and anxiety focus on the present, reducing pain perception and anxiety levels simultaneously.

Continuous Reassessment and Flexibility

Given the dynamic nature of managing multiple diagnoses, it's vital to regularly reassess the treatment plan, celebrate progress in any area, and adjust goals as needed. This iterative process acknowledges that as one issue improves or worsens, the approach to the others might also need to change.

- **Example:** If a client's efforts to reduce alcohol intake lead to a decrease in depressive symptoms, it might be appropriate to revisit and possibly intensify goals related to alcohol consumption, leveraging the improvement in mood.

Conclusion

Navigating dual diagnoses and comorbidities in MI requires a careful, client-centered approach that respects the interconnectedness of different health issues. By prioritizing issues, setting realistic goals, tailoring MI techniques, developing universal coping strategies, and maintaining flexibility, therapists can effectively support clients in managing complex health challenges, fostering hope, motivation, and a sense of agency over their well-being.

Adjusting MI techniques for different mental health disorders.

Adjusting Motivational Interviewing (MI) techniques for different mental health disorders involves tailoring conversations and strategies to meet the unique challenges and needs of each condition. This customization enhances the effectiveness of MI by ensuring that the approach resonates with the individual's experiences and struggles. Here's how MI can be adapted for various mental health disorders:

Depression

Key Adjustments: For clients with depression, who may struggle with low energy, motivation, and feelings of hopelessness, it's important to emphasize empathy and acceptance. The focus should be on setting small, achievable goals that can help build momentum and a sense of accomplishment.

- **Technique:** Use scaling questions to help clients identify small steps of progress and to explore their feelings of readiness for change in a non-overwhelming way. Highlighting any positive action or intention can be particularly motivating.

Anxiety Disorders

Key Adjustments: Clients dealing with anxiety may benefit from MI approaches that gently explore fears and worries without amplifying them. Encouraging clients to consider the benefits of change versus the costs of anxiety-driven behaviors can be helpful.

- **Technique:** Employ reflective listening to validate their experiences and concerns, while carefully guiding the conversation towards exploring how small changes could reduce anxiety levels. Incorporating discussions about coping strategies for managing anxiety can empower clients.

Substance Use Disorders

Key Adjustments: For substance use disorders, MI is particularly effective in resolving ambivalence about change. The emphasis is on exploring the pros and cons of substance use versus sobriety, in a judgment-free manner.

- **Technique:** Use the decisional balance tool to help clients weigh the benefits and drawbacks of their substance use, enhancing their motivation to pursue recovery. Eliciting change talk related to personal goals and values can foster a desire for change.

Eating Disorders

Key Adjustments: Individuals with eating disorders often face ambivalence about recovery and change. MI should be adapted to gently challenge distorted beliefs about body image and eating, without provoking resistance.

- **Technique:** Motivational enhancement strategies can help clients envision a life beyond their eating disorder, focusing on values and activities that have been overshadowed by their condition. Creating a collaborative atmosphere is key to encouraging openness about fears related to change.

PTSD and Trauma-Related Disorders

Key Adjustments: For those experiencing PTSD or trauma-related disorders, it's crucial to proceed with sensitivity to avoid retraumatization. Establishing safety and trust is paramount, with an emphasis on the client's control over the process.

- **Technique:** Utilize MI to explore the client's strengths and resilience factors, reinforcing their capacity to cope with and recover from trauma. Reflective listening becomes especially important to validate their feelings and experiences, fostering a sense of being understood and supported.

Bipolar Disorder

Key Adjustments: Working with clients who have bipolar disorder involves recognizing the impact of mood swings on motivation and perception. During manic phases, individuals may have high energy and confidence, potentially leading to unrealistic goal setting. During depressive episodes, the opposite may occur.

- **Technique:** Use MI to help the client set realistic and flexible goals, tailored to their fluctuating energy and motivation levels. During more stable periods, discuss strategies for managing both manic and depressive episodes, emphasizing the importance of adherence to treatment plans.

ADHD

Key Adjustments: Clients with Attention Deficit Hyperactivity Disorder (ADHD) may struggle with impulsivity, organization, and maintaining focus on long-term goals. MI techniques should account for these challenges, making use of clear, concise communication and focusing on immediate, achievable objectives.

- **Technique:** Break down goals into small, actionable steps and use visual aids or written summaries to reinforce key points from the conversation. Highlighting immediate benefits of change can be more motivating for individuals with ADHD, who may have a harder time visualizing distant outcomes.

Personality Disorders

Key Adjustments: For personality disorders, particularly those characterized by patterns of thinking and behavior that significantly diverge from societal expectations, MI must be adapted to address issues of trust, fear of abandonment, and identity.

- **Technique:** Establishing a strong therapeutic alliance is crucial. Use MI to explore the client's values and how they align with their goals for therapy. Reflective listening and affirmation can help validate their experiences, while gently guiding them towards considering the impact of their behaviors on their goals and relationships.

Schizophrenia and Other Psychotic Disorders

Key Adjustments: Individuals with schizophrenia or psychotic disorders may experience delusions or hallucinations that influence their perception of reality. MI in this context requires patience and a focus on building rapport and trust, emphasizing areas of the client's life that are not affected by psychosis.

- **Technique:** Focus on the client's strengths and concrete, everyday goals that can improve their quality of life. It's important to meet the client where they are, acknowledging their reality, while gently encouraging reflections on how certain changes might benefit them in practical ways.

Conclusion

Adapting MI techniques for different mental health disorders requires an understanding of the specific challenges and experiences associated with each condition. By tailoring the approach to meet the client's unique needs, therapists can more effectively engage clients in the change process, fostering motivation and resilience. The key lies in balancing empathy and support with strategic questioning and goal-setting that resonates with the client's experiences and aspirations.

Examples

The following examples illustrate how MI can be adapted to the specific challenges and needs of individuals with various mental health disorders, focusing on empathy, collaboration, and tailored strategies to foster motivation and facilitate meaningful change.

Depression

Scenario: Jamie struggles with depression and has difficulty finding motivation to engage in previously enjoyed activities.

Adjustment Example: The therapist might say, "It sounds like things you once enjoyed now feel like a chore. Can you think of one activity that might be easier to start with, something small that you've liked in the past?" This question aims to help Jamie identify a manageable step towards re-engagement, acknowledging the difficulty while fostering motivation for change.

Anxiety Disorders

Scenario: Alex experiences social anxiety and is fearful of initiating conversations at work, which hinders professional relationships.

Adjustment Example: The therapist could explore, "What's one thing you feel you could say or ask in a meeting that feels less intimidating? Let's brainstorm some low-risk ways to start engaging." This approach gently encourages Alex to consider feasible steps towards their goal, reducing the perceived risk of social interactions.

Substance Use Disorders

Scenario: Casey has recognized a need to reduce alcohol consumption but feels ambivalent about giving up social drinking.

Adjustment Example: Employing the decisional balance technique, the therapist might ask, "How does drinking fit into your life now, and what might change if you reduced your intake?" This encourages Casey to reflect on the pros and cons of their drinking behavior and its impact on life goals.

Eating Disorders

Scenario: Jordan is recovering from an eating disorder and struggles with mealtime anxiety.

Adjustment Example: The therapist might suggest, "Let's think about one meal this week where you might feel a bit more comfortable trying something new. What support would make this easier for you?" This strategy helps Jordan take small, concrete steps towards recovery, emphasizing control and support.

PTSD and Trauma-Related Disorders

Scenario: Sam, a veteran with PTSD, is hesitant to discuss traumatic experiences and avoids situations that might trigger memories.

Adjustment Example: Recognizing Sam's need for safety, the therapist might say, "It's okay to take this at your pace. What are some things you feel safe doing now that help you feel more grounded?" This prioritizes establishing safety and control over the therapeutic process.

Bipolar Disorder

Scenario: Chris, who has bipolar disorder, sets ambitious goals during manic episodes but struggles to follow through, leading to feelings of failure.

Adjustment Example: During a stable period, the therapist might discuss, "What's one goal that feels important to you, regardless of your mood? How can we break this into smaller steps that are manageable in both high and low periods?" This approach helps Chris set consistent, achievable goals.

ADHD

Scenario: Taylor, diagnosed with ADHD, finds it challenging to stay organized and meet deadlines.

Adjustment Example: The therapist could use visualization, "Imagine your workspace or calendar organized in a way that helps you feel in control. What does that look like? Let's identify one small change you can make this week to move towards that vision." This helps Taylor focus on concrete, manageable organizational strategies.

Personality Disorders

Scenario: Morgan, who has borderline personality disorder, struggles with intense emotions and fears of abandonment that impact relationships.

Adjustment Example: The therapist might explore, "When you feel overwhelmed by emotions, what's one thing that helps you feel a bit more grounded? How might we use this to help you navigate difficult moments in relationships?" This focuses on building coping skills and resilience in interpersonal contexts.

Schizophrenia and Other Psychotic Disorders

Scenario: Lee, living with schizophrenia, has goals for social engagement but is hindered by anxiety about how others perceive their symptoms.

Adjustment Example: The therapist could encourage, "What's one social activity that feels manageable to you, where you'd feel safe? Let's plan how you might approach this, including any support you might need." This supports Lee in taking gradual steps towards increased social interaction, emphasizing safety and support.

Dealing with crises and high-risk situations.

Dealing with crises and high-risk situations involves a nuanced approach that prioritizes immediate safety while respecting the client's autonomy and leveraging their intrinsic motivation for change and safety. Here's how MI principles can be applied in such scenarios:

1. Express Empathy and Validate Feelings

In a crisis, it's crucial to express empathy for the client's emotional state and validate their feelings. This helps establish a connection and trust, making it easier to navigate the situation collaboratively.

- **Example:** If a client is expressing suicidal thoughts, an MI approach would involve acknowledging the pain they're feeling without judgment, "It sounds like you're in a lot of pain right now, and things feel overwhelming."

2. Support Autonomy While Prioritizing Safety

MI emphasizes respecting the client's autonomy. Even in a crisis, it's important to involve the client in decisions about their care as much as possible, while also taking necessary steps to ensure safety.

- **Example:** For a client at risk of self-harm, you might say, "I hear how much you're hurting, and I want to support you in finding a way through this that keeps you safe. Let's talk about what we can do right now to help you feel secure."

3. Use Reflective Listening to Understand Urgency

Reflective listening is key in MI and can be particularly useful in crises to clarify the client's immediate needs and risks. It involves mirroring back what the client has said to ensure understanding and to help the client hear their own motivations for safety or change.

- **Example:** If a client is experiencing a severe panic attack, reflecting their feelings could look like, "You're feeling like everything is closing in, and it's hard to catch your breath. It's scary when it feels like you can't control what's happening."

4. Elicit and Strengthen Change Talk

Even in a high-risk situation, eliciting talk of change or safety is beneficial. Encouraging the client to verbalize their desires to remain safe or to seek help reinforces their own reasons for change.

- **Example:** In a situation where a client is contemplating leaving an abusive relationship but is afraid, eliciting change talk might involve asking, "What do you wish were different about your current situation?" or "How do you think you'd feel in a safer environment?"

5. Develop a Collaborative Safety Plan

Working together to create a safety plan can empower the client and reinforce their autonomy. This plan should include steps the client feels they can take if they feel at risk again.

- **Example:** "Let's think about some steps we can take together to help you feel safer when these feelings surface. What has helped in the past, even if only a little?"

6. Affirm Strengths and Past Successes

Highlighting the client's strengths and past successes in coping with difficult situations can bolster their confidence in their ability to handle the current crisis.

- **Example:** "You've shown incredible strength in reaching out for help today. Remember how you've gotten through tough times before. What strengths did you draw on then that you can draw on now?"

Conclusion

In dealing with crises and high-risk situations through an MI lens, the balance between ensuring immediate safety and respecting the client's autonomy is delicate but crucial. The therapist's role is to provide a supportive, empathetic presence that validates the client's experiences, encourages their autonomy in making safe choices, and leverages their internal motivations towards a path of safety and change.

Scenario: Crisis Situation Involving Suicidal Ideation

Background: Jordan, a 27-year-old software developer, has been struggling with severe depression for several months. Recently, the pressures at work have intensified, and Jordan has started to feel increasingly hopeless. Despite having a supportive partner and close friends, Jordan feels isolated and believes that others would be better off without them. Jordan has started to contemplate suicide but has not made any plans. During a therapy session, Jordan tentatively discloses these thoughts to the therapist.

Session Begins:

Therapist: "Jordan, I appreciate your courage in sharing these thoughts with me today. It sounds like things have been incredibly tough for you lately. Can you tell me a bit more about what's been going on?"

Jordan: "It's all just too much. I feel like I'm drowning, and I can't see any way out. I've started thinking that maybe my family and friends would be better off if I weren't around anymore."

Therapist Uses Reflective Listening:

Therapist: "It sounds like you're feeling overwhelmed and believe that your loved ones would be better off without you. That's a heavy burden to carry, and it's understandable that you would feel desperate for a way to ease that pain."

Assessing Immediate Risk:

Therapist: "When you have these thoughts about not being around anymore, have you thought about how you might do that?"

Jordan: "I've thought about it, but I haven't planned anything. I'm just so tired of feeling this way."

Therapist Expresses Empathy and Validates Feelings:

Therapist: "Feeling so exhausted and without hope is an incredibly difficult place to be. It's important to know that you're not alone, even if it feels that way right now. We're here together, and I'm committed to supporting you through this."

Building Autonomy and Collaboration:

Therapist: "Although things feel very dark at the moment, we can work together on small steps that might help bring some light back. It's okay if you're not sure what those steps are yet; we can explore them together. What's one thing that used to bring you a bit of comfort or peace, even if it seems small?"

Jordan: "I used to enjoy walking in the park early in the morning. It was quiet, and I felt a bit of peace then."

Developing a Safety Plan:

Therapist: "That sounds like a peaceful moment for you. Let's think about how we might incorporate those walks into your routine again, as a start. Also, it's crucial we make a plan to keep you safe, especially during moments when these thoughts become overwhelming. Who are people you trust that we can include in your safety plan?"

Jordan: "My partner and a close friend. They've been worried about me."

Therapist Affirms Strengths and Plans Follow-Up:

Therapist: "Reaching out to your partner and friend can be part of our plan. Your ability to share these feelings today shows a lot of strength. How do you feel about us meeting again in a few days to check in on how you're doing and to continue our conversation?"

Conclusion:

The therapist actively listens, validates Jordan's feelings, assesses risk, and begins collaborative planning for immediate safety and support. The approach is gentle, non-judgmental, and aimed at empowering Jordan to recognize their value and the possibilities for change, even in the midst of crisis.

Case Study Simulation 1: Handling a complex case with multiple issues.

Case Study Simulation 5: Handling a Complex Case with Multiple Issues

Background: Taylor, a 34-year-old community organizer, has been struggling with a combination of issues, including anxiety, alcohol misuse, and the recent loss of a parent, which has significantly impacted their mental health and daily functioning. Taylor feels overwhelmed by the convergence of these issues and is unsure where to begin in addressing them.

Objective: As Taylor's therapist, utilizing an integrative approach that combines elements of Motivational Interviewing (MI) with other therapeutic strategies, your goal is to help Taylor navigate these multifaceted challenges, prioritizing concerns and developing a coherent plan for moving forward.

Beginning of the Session

Therapist: "Taylor, it's clear you're juggling a lot right now, with each issue adding its own weight. It takes courage to face these challenges, and I'm here to support you through this. Could we start by talking about what feels most pressing to you at the moment?"

Taylor: "Everything just feels like too much. I don't even know where to start. My anxiety is through the roof, I'm drinking more than I should, and I can't stop thinking about my mom."

Expressing Empathy and Validating Feelings

Therapist: "You're carrying a heavy load, feeling pulled in different directions by anxiety, your grief, and trying to manage your alcohol use. It's understandable to feel lost in all of this. Let's take a step back and see if we can untangle these threads together, starting with the smallest step."

Prioritizing Issues

Therapist: "You've mentioned anxiety, alcohol use, and your grief. It might help to look at these areas one at a time. Do any of these feel like an area you're more ready or willing to explore first?"

Taylor: "Maybe my anxiety... it's always been a problem, but it's just unbearable now."

Setting a Focused Goal

Therapist: "Focusing on managing your anxiety seems like a good starting point. We can explore strategies to help you cope better. Have you noticed any particular times when your anxiety feels more manageable, even slightly?"

Taylor: "It's a bit better in the mornings or when I'm busy with work."

Developing a Strategy

Therapist: "That's useful to know. Perhaps we can build on those morning times or your work schedule to introduce a calming or grounding practice. How do you feel about trying something like mindfulness or a short breathing exercise to start your day?"

Taylor: "I could try that. I need something to help me not spiral as soon as I wake up."

Planning for Obstacles

Therapist: "Implementing a new habit comes with its ups and downs. What do you think might make it challenging to stick to this practice, and how might we address these hurdles?"

Taylor: "I might just forget or feel too rushed. Maybe I could set a reminder on my phone?"

Integrating Coping Strategies for Alcohol Misuse and Grief

Therapist: "Setting a reminder is a great idea. Also, since alcohol use and your grief are intertwined with your anxiety, let's think about how managing anxiety might impact these areas. Additionally, we can explore coping strategies that address these concerns without relying on alcohol. How does that sound?"

Taylor: "It sounds good. I'm not sure what those strategies are, but I'm willing to try."

Conclusion and Next Steps

Therapist: "We'll start with the morning mindfulness or breathing exercises and see how that influences your anxiety and overall day. We'll also work on identifying coping strategies that can support you across these challenges. Remember, this is a process, and we'll tackle it one step at a time. Let's plan to check in on how the morning routine is going in our next session and discuss any insights you might have about your alcohol use and processing your grief."

Summary

In this case study, the therapist and Taylor collaboratively identify anxiety as an initial focus area, agreeing on a manageable and specific goal to incorporate mindfulness or breathing exercises into Taylor's morning routine. The therapist ensures the plan is flexible, anticipates potential obstacles, and integrates this approach within the broader context of Taylor's alcohol misuse and grief. This integrative strategy highlights the importance of addressing complex cases with empathy, prioritizing issues, and adopting a step-by-step approach to manage multifaceted challenges.

Case Study Simulation 2: Navigating Suicidal Ideation

Background: Chris, a 29-year-old freelance writer, has been experiencing increasing feelings of isolation and hopelessness over the past few months. The pandemic has exacerbated these feelings, leading to a loss of income and a sense of purpose. Chris has started to have thoughts of suicide, believing that there is no way out of the current situation. They have not made any plans but find themselves thinking about death more frequently.

Objective: As Chris's therapist, using a compassionate and structured approach informed by principles of Crisis Intervention and Motivational Interviewing (MI), your goal is to address the immediate risk of suicidal ideation, ensure Chris's safety, and collaboratively develop a plan to navigate through this crisis.

Beginning of the Session

Therapist: "Chris, I want to thank you for being open about what you're going through. It sounds like things have been incredibly tough lately, and it takes a lot of strength to share these feelings. Can you tell me a little more about what's been on your mind?"

Chris: "I just feel stuck. Everything's collapsed around me, and I don't see any way things can get better. Sometimes, I think it would be easier if I weren't here anymore."

Assessing Immediate Risk

Therapist: "Hearing you say that you feel things might be easier if you weren't here is concerning, and I want to understand more about these thoughts. Have you thought about how you might act on these feelings?"

Chris: "Not really... I mean, I haven't planned anything. But the thoughts are there, and they scare me."

Expressing Empathy and Validating Feelings

Therapist: "It's completely understandable to feel scared when you're having these thoughts, especially during such a challenging time. You're not alone in this, and together, we can work through these feelings and find a path forward."

Creating a Safe Space and Immediate Safety Plan

Therapist: "Since these thoughts have been on your mind, let's talk about how we can keep you safe. Safety is our first priority. What are some things that might help you feel safer right now?"

Chris: "Maybe if I had someone to talk to when it gets really bad... but I don't want to burden anyone."

Building a Support System

Therapist: "Reaching out for help isn't a burden—it's a sign of strength. Let's identify a couple of people you feel comfortable reaching out to, and we can also look at some crisis resources you can access anytime. How does that sound?"

Chris: "That might help. I guess I could talk to my sister and maybe a close friend."

Developing Coping Strategies

Therapist: "Having your sister and a friend as part of your support system is a great step. We can also work on some coping strategies you can use when these thoughts arise. For example, engaging in an activity that keeps your hands and mind busy can be a good distraction. What activities have helped in the past?"

Chris: "I used to enjoy drawing. It helped me focus on something else."

Planning for Follow-Up

Therapist: "Drawing sounds like a wonderful coping strategy. Let's plan for you to spend some time drawing each day, and we'll also schedule regular check-ins to talk about how you're doing. Your safety and well-being are paramount, and I'm here to support you through this."

Conclusion

The therapist works with Chris to assess the risk of suicide, validates their feelings, and emphasizes the importance of safety and support. By identifying immediate support options and engaging coping mechanisms, such as drawing, the therapist helps Chris begin to see alternative paths forward. Regular follow-up appointments are scheduled to provide ongoing support, monitor Chris's safety, and continue exploring underlying issues contributing to their suicidal ideation.

Summary

In this case study, addressing Chris's suicidal ideation involves a careful balance of immediate risk assessment, empathy, building a support network, and empowering Chris with coping strategies. The therapist's approach is grounded in validating Chris's experience, enhancing their safety, and fostering hope and resilience during a vulnerable time.

Chapter 7: Real-time Feedback and Skill Enhancement

Incorporating feedback into practice.

Incorporating feedback into therapeutic practice is a cornerstone of professional growth, client satisfaction, and improved therapeutic outcomes. It involves actively seeking, receiving, and integrating feedback from clients and peers into your approach and methodologies. This process can enhance the therapeutic alliance, adapt interventions to better meet client needs, and refine your skills as a therapist. Here's a guide on how to effectively incorporate feedback into practice:

1. Create a Feedback-Friendly Environment

- **Strategy:** Make it clear to clients from the outset that their feedback is valuable and welcome. This can be done by explicitly asking for feedback at various points in the therapeutic process, such as after introducing a new intervention or at the end of a session.

- **Example:** "I'd love to hear how you felt about today's session and if there's anything you think could be more helpful for you going forward."

2. Use Structured Feedback Tools

- **Strategy:** Employ standardized feedback tools or questionnaires designed to measure therapeutic outcomes and the client-therapist relationship. These tools can provide objective data on areas of strength and those needing improvement.

- **Example:** Implementing the Session Rating Scale (SRS) or the Outcome Rating Scale (ORS) at the end of sessions to get regular feedback on the therapeutic alliance and client satisfaction.

3. Peer Consultation and Supervision

- **Strategy:** Regularly discuss cases (while maintaining confidentiality) with peers or a supervisor to gain different perspectives and feedback on your therapeutic approach, particularly for complex cases or when feeling stuck.

- **Example:** Bringing a challenging case to a supervision session or peer consultation group to explore alternative strategies and receive constructive feedback on your approach.

4. Reflective Practice

- **Strategy:** Engage in regular self-reflection on your practice, considering the feedback received from clients and peers. Reflect on what worked well, what didn't, and why, to identify areas for personal and professional growth.

- **Example:** Keeping a reflective journal where you note feedback from clients and peers, your observations, and action plans for incorporating this feedback into your practice.

5. Professional Development

- **Strategy:** Use feedback as a guide for continuing education and professional development opportunities. Seek out workshops, courses, or reading materials that address areas where you wish to grow or strengthen your skills.

- **Example:** If feedback indicates a need to improve skills in managing transference and countertransference, attending a workshop on psychoanalytic approaches to therapy could be beneficial.

6. Implement Changes and Communicate Back

- **Strategy:** When feasible and appropriate, make changes based on the feedback received and let your clients know how their input has influenced your practice. This can reinforce the therapeutic alliance and show clients that their perspectives are valued and respected.

- **Example:** "Based on what you've shared with me about preferring a more structured approach to our sessions, I've incorporated a brief agenda at the beginning to outline what we'll cover today."

7. Monitor the Impact of Changes

- **Strategy:** After incorporating feedback and making adjustments, closely monitor the impact of these changes on therapeutic outcomes and client satisfaction. This ongoing evaluation can inform further adjustments and fine-tuning.

- **Example:** Following the introduction of more structured session agendas, checking in with the client after a few sessions to assess how this change is impacting their experience and the therapeutic work.

Conclusion

Incorporating feedback into therapeutic practice is a dynamic process that requires openness, flexibility, and a commitment to ongoing learning and improvement. By valuing and acting on feedback from clients and peers, therapists can enhance their effectiveness, adaptability, and ultimately, the quality of care they provide.

Self-assessment and continuous improvement

Self-assessment and continuous improvement are crucial for professionals in any field, especially in therapeutic practices where the quality of the interaction can significantly impact client outcomes. Here are several techniques that can help therapists and similar professionals engage in self-assessment and foster continuous improvement:

1. Reflective Journaling

- **Description:** Keeping a daily or weekly journal where you reflect on your sessions, your feelings, reactions, and the decisions you made. This can help you identify patterns in your practice, areas of strength, and areas for growth.

- **Implementation:** After each session, take a few minutes to jot down key takeaways, what you felt went well, what could have been better, and any emotional responses you experienced.

2. Feedback Loops

- **Description:** Actively seeking feedback from clients, peers, and supervisors. Feedback can provide direct insight into areas of effectiveness and those requiring improvement.

- **Implementation:** Use standardized tools like the Session Rating Scale (SRS) for client feedback, and establish regular peer supervision sessions where you can receive constructive criticism.

3. Video or Audio Recording Sessions

- **Description:** With consent, recording sessions to review your therapeutic techniques, client interactions, and moments of breakthrough or resistance.

- **Implementation:** Periodically record sessions and review them alone or with a supervisor to analyze your therapeutic approach, questioning techniques, and non-verbal communication.

4. Goal Setting and Monitoring

- **Description:** Setting specific, measurable, achievable, relevant, and time-bound (SMART) goals for your professional development and monitoring your progress towards these goals.

- **Implementation:** Set a goal to improve a particular skill or area of knowledge, such as becoming more proficient in a therapeutic approach, and track your progress through continued education, practice, and reflection.

5. Professional Development Activities

- **Description:** Engaging in continuous learning through workshops, seminars, courses, and reading relevant literature.

- **Implementation:** Identify areas for growth and seek out professional development opportunities in those areas.

After completing an activity, reflect on how you can integrate new knowledge or skills into your practice.

6. Peer Consultation Groups

- **Description:** Participating in or forming a peer consultation group to discuss cases (while maintaining confidentiality), share experiences, and get insights from colleagues.

- **Implementation:** Meet regularly with a group of peers to discuss challenges, share successes, and offer each other feedback and support.

7. Self-Care Practices

- **Description:** Engaging in regular self-care to prevent burnout and maintain emotional and physical well-being, which is essential for effective practice.

- **Implementation:** Incorporate activities into your routine that help manage stress, such as exercise, meditation, hobbies, and ensuring a healthy work-life balance.

8. Mindfulness and Self-observation

- **Description:** Practicing mindfulness to become more aware of your own thoughts, feelings, and reactions during therapy sessions.

- **Implementation:** Develop a mindfulness practice that allows you to observe your reactions and emotions without judgment, both during sessions and in your daily life.

9. Utilizing Technology and Apps

- **Description:** Making use of apps and technology designed for professional development, such as mindfulness apps, e-learning platforms, or feedback tools.

- **Implementation:** Explore apps and platforms that offer relevant content for therapists, such as case management simulations, mindfulness exercises, or platforms offering courses on specific therapeutic techniques.

Conclusion

Self-assessment and continuous improvement are ongoing processes that require dedication, curiosity, and a willingness to be vulnerable and open to change. By implementing these techniques, therapists and other professionals can ensure they are providing the best possible care to their clients while also attending to their own growth and well-being.

Example

Background

Dr. Elena is a clinical psychologist specializing in cognitive-behavioral therapy (CBT) for adults with anxiety disorders. Despite her years of experience, she remains committed to improving her practice and staying updated with the latest research and techniques in her field.

Reflective Journaling

Implementation: After each therapy session, Dr. Elena spends 10 minutes reflecting on the session's dynamics. She notes any moments where the client seemed particularly engaged or resistant and reflects on her interventions' effectiveness. She questions whether alternative strategies might have been more beneficial in certain situations.

Feedback Loops

Implementation: Dr. Elena implements the Session Rating Scale (SRS) at the end of each session, asking her clients to rate the session's aspects, such as the therapeutic relationship, goals and topics, approach or method, and overall session. She reviews this feedback weekly to identify any patterns or areas for improvement.

Video Recording Sessions

Implementation: Once a month, with her client's consent, Dr. Elena records a session. She later reviews this recording, focusing on her use of CBT techniques, her non-verbal communication, and how she handles moments of resistance. She often shares these recordings with a trusted colleague for an external perspective.

Goal Setting and Monitoring

Implementation: Dr. Elena sets a goal to enhance her expertise in treating anxiety disorders with exposure therapy, a subset of CBT. She tracks her progress by attending workshops, reading current literature, and gradually incorporating exposure therapy techniques into her practice with suitable clients.

Professional Development Activities

Implementation: Dr. Elena attends an annual CBT conference, participates in online webinars, and subscribes to professional journals. After each learning activity, she integrates at least one new insight or technique into her practice and discusses its applicability and effectiveness in her peer consultation group.

Peer Consultation Groups

Implementation: Bi-weekly, Dr. Elena meets with a group of psychologists where they discuss challenging cases (while maintaining confidentiality), share insights, and provide feedback on each other's therapeutic approaches. These sessions are invaluable for gaining new perspectives and strategies.

Self-Care Practices

Implementation: Understanding the importance of self-care, Dr. Elena practices yoga three times a week and engages in a mindfulness meditation session daily. These practices help her manage stress, maintain her well-being, and approach her client sessions with a clear, focused mind.

Mindfulness and Self-Observation

Implementation: Dr. Elena practices mindfulness during her sessions, staying present and attuned to her reactions and feelings. This helps her remain empathetic and effectively respond to her clients' needs while also recognizing her emotional boundaries.

Utilizing Technology and Apps

Implementation: Dr. Elena uses an app designed for mental health professionals that features regular updates on research, technique tutorials, and community forums. This app allows her to stay informed about advancements in her field and connect with other professionals for advice and support.

Conclusion

Through these diverse techniques, Dr. Elena exemplifies a commitment to self-assessment and continuous improvement. By reflecting on her practice, seeking feedback, staying informed about new research, and prioritizing her well-being, she ensures that she provides the highest quality care to her clients while also fostering her professional growth.

Supervision and peer feedback

Utilizing supervision and peer feedback is an essential part of professional development in therapeutic practices. These avenues provide critical insights, support, and guidance that can enhance clinical skills, therapeutic relationships, and overall effectiveness. Here's how to make the most of supervision and peer feedback:

Engaging in Supervision

1. Be Open and Prepared

- **Approach:** Come to supervision sessions prepared with specific cases, questions, or themes you want to explore. Openness to feedback is crucial; view it as an opportunity for growth rather than criticism.

- **Example:** Before supervision, Dr. Lee prepares a list of challenging moments from recent sessions, including a time when they felt stuck with a client's resistance to change. They are ready to discuss these openly, seeking insights and strategies.

2. Reflective Practice

- **Approach:** Use supervision as a space for reflective practice. Discuss your thoughts, feelings, and reactions to therapy sessions and how these impact your work. Reflecting on your practice helps identify areas for growth and development.

- **Example:** Dr. Lee shares their feelings of frustration and doubt when a client does not seem to progress. Through reflection, they explore how these feelings might affect their approach to therapy and client interaction.

3. Actionable Feedback

- **Approach:** Seek specific, actionable feedback rather than general comments. This type of feedback can directly inform and improve your practice.

- **Example:** Instead of asking, "How am I doing?" Dr. Lee asks, "Can you give me specific feedback on how I handled the client's disclosure in our last session?"

Utilizing Peer Feedback

1. Peer Consultation Groups

- **Approach:** Participate in or form a peer consultation group. These groups offer diverse perspectives and can be a source of support, validation, and challenge.

- **Example:** Dr. Lee meets monthly with a peer group where they present cases in a confidential setting, offering and receiving feedback on therapeutic techniques, client management, and self-care practices.

2. Reciprocal Observation

- **Approach:** Arrange reciprocal observation sessions with peers where you observe each other's sessions (with client consent) and provide feedback. This can offer new insights into your therapeutic style and client interactions.

- **Example:** Dr. Lee and a colleague agree to observe each other's sessions. After the observation, they discuss their observations and provide feedback on specific interventions and client engagement strategies.

3. Specificity and Constructiveness

- **Approach:** When giving and receiving peer feedback, be as specific and constructive as possible. Focus on observable behaviors and outcomes, and suggest alternative strategies or approaches.

- **Example:** After observing Dr. Lee's session, a peer provides specific feedback: "When the client expressed feeling stuck, I noticed you quickly offered solutions. Perhaps spending more time exploring their feelings of being stuck might help them feel more understood and open up further. Have you considered using more reflective listening in that moment?"

Integrating Feedback into Practice

1. Develop an Action Plan

- **Approach:** After receiving feedback, develop a concrete action plan to integrate the insights and suggestions into your practice. Identify specific steps, strategies, or techniques you will try, and set timelines for implementation and review.

- **Example:** Based on feedback about needing to enhance reflective listening, Dr. Lee decides to focus on this skill in the next month, setting a goal to incorporate at least three reflective statements in each session and journaling about the outcomes.

2. Continuous Learning

- **Approach:** View feedback as part of an ongoing learning process. Engage in continuous education, workshops, and reading to address the areas identified through feedback.

- **Example:** To improve their understanding and implementation of reflective listening, Dr. Lee enrolls in a workshop focused on advanced listening skills and reads current articles on the topic to enhance their knowledge and application in therapy sessions.

3. Follow-Up and Re-evaluation

- **Approach:** After implementing changes based on supervision and peer feedback, seek follow-up feedback to evaluate the effectiveness of the changes and make further adjustments as needed.

- **Example:** After focusing on reflective listening for a month, Dr. Lee requests feedback from their supervisor and peers again to assess progress and determine if clients have noticed a change in their experience of being heard and understood.

Creating a Feedback Culture

1. Promote a Culture of Feedback

- **Approach:** Foster an environment where giving and receiving feedback is a normal, valued part of professional development. This can reduce defensiveness and promote a growth mindset.

- **Example:** Dr. Lee encourages feedback within their peer consultation group, emphasizing the importance of constructive criticism and celebrating the application of feedback in practice.

2. Self-Compassion and Resilience

- **Approach:** Practice self-compassion and resilience in the face of feedback that may be challenging to hear. Recognize that growth often comes from addressing difficult areas.

- **Example:** When receiving feedback that highlights a need for improvement, Dr. Lee reminds themselves that growth is an ongoing process and that identifying areas for improvement is a strength, not a weakness.

Conclusion

Effectively utilizing supervision and peer feedback involves preparation, openness, specificity, and a commitment to integrating insights into practice. By approaching feedback as a valuable resource for learning and growth, therapists can continually enhance their skills, therapeutic relationships, and ultimately, client outcomes.

Simulation: Interactive feedback session based on recorded sessions.

Background: Dr. Alex Thompson, a therapist specializing in anxiety disorders, has been working to improve their therapeutic techniques and client engagement. Dr. Thompson has recorded a session with a client, "Jordan," who has consented to the recording for educational purposes, aiming to enhance the therapeutic process. The recorded session focuses on exploring Jordan's triggers for anxiety and discussing coping strategies.

Objective: Dr. Thompson participates in an interactive feedback session with their supervisor, Dr. Lena Martinez, to review the recorded session, identify strengths, areas for improvement, and develop an action plan for enhancing therapeutic skills.

Setting: The feedback session takes place in a quiet, confidential meeting room, with both Dr. Thompson and Dr. Martinez having watched the recorded session prior to the meeting.

Dr. Martinez: "Alex, thank you for sharing this session. It's a valuable tool for reflection and growth. Let's start with your initial thoughts. How did you feel the session went?"

Dr. Thompson: "I felt it went well overall, but I'm aware there's room for improvement, especially in how I engage Jordan in exploring their anxiety triggers more deeply."

Dr. Martinez: "I agree, you established a supportive environment. Let's dive into some specifics. I noticed a moment where Jordan mentioned feeling anxious in social settings, and you quickly moved on to coping strategies. Can you tell me more about that choice?"

Dr. Thompson: "Looking back, I think I might have moved too quickly because I wanted to provide Jordan with immediate relief. I see now that exploring those feelings more thoroughly could have provided deeper insights."

Dr. Martinez: "That's a valuable observation. Exploring emotions can indeed offer deeper healing. Let's consider how we might approach a similar situation in the future. What are your thoughts?"

Dr. Thompson: "Perhaps I could use more open-ended questions to encourage Jordan to express more about their feelings regarding social settings, showing more curiosity about their experience."

Dr. Martinez: "Exactly, open-ended questions can be powerful. I also noticed you used reflective listening effectively in several parts of the session. For example, when Jordan talked about their work stress, your reflections helped them articulate their thoughts more clearly. That's a strength to build on."

Dr. Thompson: "Thank you, I've been working on that. I'll continue to focus on reflective listening and apply it more consistently throughout the sessions."

Dr. Martinez: "Let's talk about the transition to coping strategies. You introduced a breathing technique, which Jordan seemed receptive to. How do you feel about the timing and integration of that technique?"

Dr. Thompson: "I thought it was a good moment to introduce a practical tool, but I wonder if I could have first validated Jordan's feelings about their social anxiety more before transitioning."

Dr. Martinez: "That's an insightful reflection. Validating feelings can indeed reinforce the therapeutic alliance and make the introduction of coping strategies feel more attuned to the client's needs. Maybe next time, you could try a brief validation, like 'It sounds like social situations bring up a lot of anxiety for you, which must be really challenging. There's a technique I think could help, but I want to make sure you feel fully heard first.' How does that sound?"

Dr. Thompson: "That sounds great. It maintains the flow and ensures Jordan feels understood. I'll incorporate that approach."

Dr. Martinez: "Wonderful. Now, considering the entire session, what's one goal you'd like to set for your next sessions with Jordan or similar clients?"

Dr. Thompson: "I want to improve my ability to balance exploring emotions with providing coping strategies. Specifically, I aim to use more open-ended questions and ensure clients feel heard before moving on to solutions."

Dr. Martinez: "That's a solid goal, Alex. Balancing exploration with solution-focused interventions is key to effective therapy. Let's plan a follow-up in a few weeks to discuss your progress and any new insights. Also, consider journaling about your experiences as you work on this goal. It could provide valuable reflections for our next meeting."

Dr. Thompson: "I will, and thank you, Lena, for the constructive feedback and guidance. I appreciate the support and the opportunity to learn and grow in my practice."

Dr. Martinez: "Of course, Alex. Remember, the goal of feedback is not only to identify areas for improvement but also to recognize and build on your strengths. You're doing important work, and I'm here to support you in continuing to develop your skills."

Conclusion: The feedback session concludes with Dr. Thompson feeling supported and motivated, armed with specific strategies for improvement and an action plan for their professional development. Dr. Martinez has successfully provided a balanced mix of positive reinforcement and constructive feedback, emphasizing the importance of continuous learning and growth in therapeutic practice.

This simulation underscores the importance of effective communication, the value of reflective practice, and the role of supervision in professional development. By engaging in such detailed feedback sessions, therapists can enhance their skills, deepen their understanding of client needs, and improve therapeutic outcomes.

Chapter 8: Advanced Applications of MI

Integrating MI with other therapeutic approaches

Integrating Motivational Interviewing (MI) with other therapeutic approaches, such as Cognitive Behavioral Therapy (CBT) and Dialectical Behavior Therapy (DBT), can enhance the effectiveness of treatment by addressing motivation and resistance, and by providing structured strategies for change. Here's how MI can be harmoniously integrated with these approaches:

MI and CBT

Integration Strategy:

- **Initial Engagement:** Use MI in the early stages of therapy to explore ambivalence and enhance motivation for change. This sets a collaborative tone for the therapeutic relationship, crucial for the more structured CBT that follows.

- **Setting Goals:** Once motivation is established, transition to CBT to set specific, measurable goals. The client's increased readiness for change can make CBT interventions more effective.

- **Combining Techniques:** Incorporate MI techniques when introducing CBT strategies. For example, when discussing cognitive distortions, use MI to explore the client's thoughts and feelings about these patterns without judgment, enhancing their openness to cognitive restructuring.

- **Addressing Resistance:** When resistance to CBT homework or exercises arises, revert to MI techniques to explore the client's hesitations and reinforce their autonomy and competence.

Example Scenario: A client is initially hesitant to engage in exposure therapy for social anxiety. The therapist uses MI to explore the client's fears and desires related to social interactions, building motivation. As the client becomes more open to change, the therapist introduces CBT-based exposure exercises, using MI to reinforce the client's successes and navigate any resistance to specific tasks.

MI and DBT

Integration Strategy:

- **Enhancing Commitment:** MI can be particularly useful in the commitment phase of DBT, helping clients commit to the treatment and to working on distress tolerance, emotion regulation, and interpersonal effectiveness skills.

- **Validating Emotions:** MI's emphasis on empathy and validation complements DBT's focus on validating the client's experiences and emotions, creating a supportive environment for exploring difficult emotions and behaviors.

- **Targeting Ambivalence:** Use MI to address ambivalence towards behavioral changes that DBT aims to achieve, such as reducing self-harm behaviors or improving communication in relationships.

- **Skill Generalization:** MI techniques can be used to reinforce the application of DBT skills in real-life situations, encouraging clients to reflect on their experiences and reinforcing their confidence in using these skills independently.

Example Scenario: A client struggles with emotional dysregulation and self-harm. Through MI, the therapist helps the client articulate their mixed feelings about self-harm and its impact on their life, building readiness to try new coping strategies. As the client shows willingness to change, the therapist integrates DBT skills training, focusing on emotion regulation and distress tolerance, while continuing to use MI to reinforce progress and work through setbacks.

General Considerations for Integration

- **Seamless Transition:** Effective integration requires a seamless transition between MI and other approaches. Therapists should be fluent in both MI and the other therapeutic models to appropriately weave them together based on the client's needs.

- **Client-Centered Approach:** Regardless of the therapeutic model, maintaining a client-centered approach is key. The integration should always honor the client's pace, values, and readiness for change.

- **Continuous Assessment:** Regularly assess the client's response to the integrated approach, being prepared to adjust the balance between MI and other strategies to meet the evolving needs of the client.

Conclusion

Integrating MI with CBT, DBT, or other therapeutic approaches can provide a comprehensive framework for facilitating change. By combining MI's focus on motivation and ambivalence with the structured strategies and skills offered by CBT and DBT, therapists can offer a nuanced, adaptable, and highly effective treatment.

Advanced Integration Techniques for MI with Other Therapies

Integrating Motivational Interviewing (MI) with other therapeutic models like CBT and DBT not only enhances client engagement but also ensures a more holistic approach to treatment. Below are more advanced techniques and considerations for effective integration across different stages of therapy:

During Assessment and Goal Setting

- **Dual Focus on Motivation and Goals:** Utilize MI to explore the client's values and motivations in depth during the initial assessment phase. This understanding can then inform the goal-setting process in CBT or the identification of target behaviors in DBT, ensuring goals are intrinsically motivating to the client.

- **Example:** In a session focusing on depression, after using MI to understand the client's personal values around relationships and self-image, a therapist can guide the goal-setting process in CBT to prioritize improving social interactions and enhancing self-esteem.

Enhancing Skill Acquisition

- **MI to Overcome Learning Barriers:** When introducing new skills or coping strategies, whether from CBT (e.g., cognitive restructuring) or DBT (e.g., mindfulness exercises), use MI to address any reluctance or perceived barriers to learning these skills.

- **Example:** If a client is skeptical about the benefits of mindfulness exercises from DBT, an MI approach can help explore this skepticism, relate the exercises to the client's personal goals or values, and gradually build willingness to engage.

During the Action Phase

- **Reinforcing Progress with MI:** As clients begin to apply new skills or change behaviors, use MI to reinforce progress, highlighting how these changes align with their broader goals and values. This can increase intrinsic motivation to maintain these changes.

- **Example:** When a client successfully employs a new coping strategy learned in CBT to manage anxiety triggers, the therapist uses MI to reinforce this progress, linking it back to the client's desire for greater independence and control over their life.

Addressing Setbacks

- **Combining Approaches to Navigate Setbacks:** Use MI to navigate setbacks empathetically, exploring the client's feelings about the setback and reinforcing their autonomy and capacity for resilience. Follow this with targeted CBT or DBT strategies to analyze the setback and plan for future success.

- **Example:** After a relapse in substance use, the therapist first uses MI to address feelings of guilt and failure, emphasizing the client's strengths. Then, they employ CBT strategies to examine the thoughts and situations that led to the relapse, planning more effective coping strategies for the future.

Maintenance and Relapse Prevention

- **Long-Term Motivation and Planning:** As clients move into maintenance phases or work on relapse prevention, continue to use MI to explore and reinforce long-term motivations for wellness. Integrate this with specific CBT or DBT strategies for recognizing early warning signs and implementing coping strategies.

- **Example:** For a client in recovery from addiction, combine MI discussions about the client's vision for their future with DBT skills for managing cravings and emotional distress, creating a comprehensive relapse prevention plan.

Continuous Professional Development

- **Therapist Growth:** Therapists should pursue ongoing training and supervision in both MI and the specific therapeutic models they integrate (CBT, DBT, etc.) to stay abreast of best practices and enhance their integration skills.

- **Example:** Participate in interdisciplinary workshops that focus on the integration of MI with CBT or DBT, and seek supervision from experienced practitioners who specialize in these integrative approaches.

Conclusion

The integration of MI with other therapeutic approaches requires thoughtful application, flexibility, and a commitment to client-centered practice. By skillfully combining the strengths of MI with the structured interventions of CBT and DBT, therapists can offer nuanced and effective support that resonates deeply with clients' experiences and aspirations for change.

Adapting MI for diverse populations

Adapting Motivational Interviewing (MI) for diverse populations involves recognizing and respecting cultural, ethnic, and individual differences that influence clients' values, beliefs, and behaviors. Cultural considerations are crucial for ensuring MI is effective and respectful, fostering a therapeutic environment where all clients feel understood and valued. Here are strategies for adapting MI with an emphasis on cultural sensitivity:

Understanding Cultural Context

Approach: Gain knowledge about the cultural backgrounds of your clients to better understand their worldviews, communication styles, and values. This awareness can guide your use of MI, ensuring that your approach aligns with the client's cultural context.

- **Example:** If a therapist is working with a client from a culture that values community and collective decision-making, the therapist might emphasize how changes the client is considering could benefit not just the individual but also their family and community.

Respecting Communication Styles

Approach: Adapt your communication to match the client's preferred style, which may be influenced by their cultural background. This includes adjusting the pace of the conversation, the directness of questioning, and the use of silence.

- **Example:** In cultures where direct confrontation is avoided, a therapist might use more reflective listening and indirect questioning to explore ambivalence, rather than directly challenging the client's statements.

Incorporating Cultural Values into Goals

Approach: Work with clients to set goals that are meaningful within their cultural context. Understanding and incorporating clients' values can enhance their motivation for change by ensuring that goals are relevant and culturally congruent.

- **Example:** For a client whose culture places a high value on familial obligations, goals related to improving personal health or reducing substance use might be framed in terms of being able to fulfill family roles more effectively.

Using Culturally Relevant Metaphors and Examples

Approach: Employ metaphors, stories, and examples that are culturally relevant to the client. This can make MI more engaging and relatable, helping to bridge cultural gaps between the therapist and client.

- **Example:** A therapist working with a Native American client might use storytelling, a traditional teaching method in many Native cultures, to illustrate concepts related to change and growth.

Addressing Cultural Mistrust and Barriers

Approach: Acknowledge and address any mistrust or barriers that may arise from historical or personal experiences of discrimination or marginalization. Demonstrating awareness and sensitivity to these issues can strengthen the therapeutic alliance.

- **Example:** A therapist might openly acknowledge the systemic barriers a client of color faces in accessing healthcare, including mental health services, and discuss how they can work together to navigate these challenges.

Engaging with Cultural Strengths and Resources

Approach: Identify and build on cultural strengths and resources that can support the client's journey toward change. Every culture has unique strengths, such as community support networks, traditional healing practices, or spiritual beliefs, that can be integrated into the therapeutic process.

- **Example:** For a client who draws strength from their spiritual faith, integrating prayer or other spiritual practices into their coping strategies might be explored as part of the MI process.

Training and Supervision

Approach: Seek ongoing cultural competence training and supervision to continually improve your ability to work effectively with diverse populations. Staying informed about cultural issues and reflecting on your own cultural biases are key components of professional development.

- **Example:** Participating in workshops on cultural humility and seeking supervision from therapists experienced in cross-cultural practice can enhance a therapist's ability to adapt MI in culturally sensitive ways.

Collaborative Goal Setting

Approach: Collaboratively set goals with clients that not only respect but also leverage their cultural identities and resources.

This collaborative process ensures that goals are both culturally relevant and aligned with clients' personal values and community norms.

- **Example:** A therapist working with an immigrant client might explore goals that consider the challenges of acculturation and identity. For instance, finding ways to maintain cultural traditions while navigating the stressors of adapting to a new culture could be an important therapeutic goal.

Language and Communication

Approach: Be mindful of language barriers and the role of non-verbal communication in different cultures. When necessary, employ the services of a professional interpreter who is not only fluent in the client's language but also knowledgeable about cultural nuances.

- **Example:** In sessions with clients who speak a different language, a therapist ensures that an interpreter is present and takes the time to understand the client's non-verbal cues, which may carry significant cultural meaning.

Exploring Cultural Identity

Approach: Use MI to explore and affirm the client's cultural identity as part of the therapeutic process. Understanding how clients perceive their cultural identity can provide insights into their values and how these influence their motivation for change.

- **Example:** A therapist might ask reflective questions that encourage clients to share how their cultural identity influences their view of health, wellness, and behavior change, integrating these insights into the motivation for therapy.

Handling Cultural Conflicts

Approach: When cultural conflicts arise, such as intergenerational tensions within immigrant families or conflicts between personal and cultural values, use MI to navigate these conflicts sensitively. MI can help clients explore these tensions and find personally meaningful ways to address them.

- **Example:** For a young adult from a traditional background struggling with expectations around marriage, a therapist could use MI to help them articulate their desires and fears, facilitating a dialogue about balancing personal choices with cultural expectations.

Continuous Cultural Competency Development

Approach: Recognize that cultural competency is not a destination but a continuous journey. Therapists should engage in lifelong learning and self-reflection to understand the diverse cultural backgrounds of their clients better and to challenge their own assumptions and biases.

- **Example:** A therapist regularly attends cultural competency seminars and participates in discussion groups with colleagues to reflect on how cultural issues impact therapy, ensuring their approach remains respectful and responsive to diverse client needs.

Conclusion

Integrating cultural considerations into Motivational Interviewing practices enriches the therapeutic process, making it more inclusive and effective for clients from diverse backgrounds. By actively engaging with clients' cultural contexts, therapists can better support their journey towards change, ensuring that therapy is a culturally safe space where all clients feel valued and understood. This approach not only enhances the efficacy of MI but also contributes to a broader understanding and appreciation of cultural diversity within the therapeutic community.

Telehealth and digital platforms for MI

The adaptation of Motivational Interviewing (MI) to telehealth and digital platforms has become increasingly relevant, especially in the context of the global shift towards more remote and accessible healthcare services. Delivering MI through telehealth poses unique challenges but also offers opportunities for innovation and expanded reach. Here's how MI principles can be effectively applied in a digital context:

1. Maintaining Client Engagement

- **Challenge:** Engaging clients and building rapport can be more challenging through a screen, where non-verbal cues are harder to read, and the sense of presence may be diminished.

- **Solution:** Use clear, expressive communication and be intentional about showing attentiveness through verbal nods and summarizations. Regularly check in with the client about their comfort with the format and any adjustments that might enhance their experience.

2. Creating a Safe and Confidential Space

- **Challenge:** Ensuring privacy and confidentiality can be more complex in telehealth, where sessions might be conducted in less controlled environments.

- **Solution:** Prior to starting MI sessions via telehealth, provide clients with guidance on creating a private space for their sessions. Discuss and agree on protocols for ensuring privacy from both ends, including the use of secure, encrypted platforms for communication.

3. Adapting MI Techniques for Digital Delivery

- **Challenge:** Some MI techniques, particularly those reliant on non-verbal communication and subtle cues, may need adjustment when delivered via telehealth.

- **Solution:** Adapt MI techniques to emphasize verbal reflections and affirmations. Increase the use of open-ended questions and reflective listening to compensate for the reduced ability to rely on non-verbal cues. Utilize chat features for clients to type out thoughts they might find difficult to express verbally.

4. Leveraging Digital Tools

- **Opportunity:** Digital platforms offer unique tools and resources that can enhance MI practice, such as shared screens for reviewing progress, digital worksheets, and apps for tracking goals and changes.

- **Implementation:** Integrate the use of digital tools within MI sessions, such as sharing educational resources, interactive worksheets, or applications that allow clients to monitor their progress towards their goals, enhancing their engagement and motivation.

5. Addressing Digital Literacy and Access

- **Challenge:** Clients vary in their comfort and ability to use digital platforms, and some may have limited access to the necessary technology.

- **Solution:** Provide clear instructions and support for using telehealth platforms, considering the client's level of digital literacy. Offer alternatives where necessary, such as telephone sessions, and work with clients to find the most accessible and comfortable format for them.

6. Ensuring Continuity of Care

- **Opportunity:** Telehealth can improve the continuity of care by offering greater flexibility and reducing barriers to access, such as transportation or mobility issues.

- **Implementation:** Use telehealth as an opportunity to maintain regular contact with clients, scheduling follow-ups and check-ins with greater flexibility. This can help sustain motivation and engagement in clients who might otherwise struggle to attend in-person sessions.

7. Training and Supervision

- **Necessity:** Therapists need training and support to adapt MI techniques to telehealth effectively, ensuring fidelity to MI principles while navigating the nuances of digital delivery.

- **Implementation:** Engage in professional development opportunities focused on delivering psychological therapies, including MI, through telehealth. Seek supervision and feedback on telehealth sessions to refine skills and strategies for digital engagement.

Conclusion

The integration of Motivational Interviewing within telehealth and digital platforms requires thoughtful adaptation and creativity but offers a valuable avenue for reaching and engaging clients. By leveraging technology effectively, therapists can maintain the client-centered, empathetic essence of MI, ensuring that the therapeutic principles of MI are preserved and even enhanced in a digital format.

Case Study Simulation 1: Applying MI in a culturally sensitive manner

Background: Amina is a 40-year-old woman who recently immigrated to the United States from Nigeria with her two children and husband. She has been experiencing significant stress and anxiety due to the cultural transition, financial pressures, and her efforts to maintain her cultural identity while adapting to a new society. Amina seeks therapy to manage her stress and anxiety but expresses concern about being understood by someone outside her cultural background.

Objective: As Amina's therapist, using Motivational Interviewing (MI) in a culturally sensitive manner, your goal is to help Amina explore her feelings about her current situation, enhance her motivation to find coping strategies that respect her cultural identity, and support her in navigating the challenges of acculturation.

Beginning of the Session

Therapist: "Amina, thank you for sharing your story with me. It sounds like you're navigating many changes and facing some really challenging situations. I want to acknowledge the strength it takes to manage all this, especially while keeping your cultural values and traditions alive. How do you feel about the changes you and your family are going through?"

Expressing Empathy and Validating Feelings

Therapist: "It's completely understandable to feel stressed and anxious given everything you're dealing with. Moving to a new country and adapting to a different culture can be incredibly challenging. Your feelings are valid, and it's important to me that we find ways to address them that feel true to who you are."

Exploring Ambivalence

Therapist: "You mentioned wanting to maintain your cultural identity while adapting to life here. That's a significant balance to strike. Can you tell me more about what aspects of your culture are most important to you, and how you're finding the process of adapting to a new environment?"

Reflecting Cultural Values in Goals

Therapist: "From what you've shared, it sounds like family and community play a big role in your life. How can we use these values as a foundation to explore coping strategies for your stress and anxiety? Are there practices from your culture that have helped you in the past that we can integrate into our approach?"

Addressing Cultural Mistrust and Barriers

Therapist: "I understand that talking about personal challenges with someone from a different cultural background might bring up some concerns for you. I'm here to learn from you about your experiences and perspective. What can I do to make this space feel safer and more understanding of your cultural needs?"

Engaging with Cultural Strengths and Resources

Therapist: "You have a rich cultural heritage that can be a source of strength during this time. Let's explore how we can draw on your cultural practices, community resources, or any aspects of your faith or traditions that could support your well-being."

Conclusion and Next Steps

Therapist: "Amina, it's clear you have a strong connection to your cultural roots, and those roots can help us navigate the challenges you're facing. For our next session, I'd like you to think about a time when your cultural practices helped you overcome a difficult situation. We can use those insights to build strategies that honor your identity and support you in this transition."

Summary

This case study simulation emphasizes the importance of applying MI in a culturally sensitive manner, recognizing and validating the client's cultural background, and using it as a strength in therapy. The therapist's approach is respectful, empathetic, and tailored to Amina's unique experiences and values, fostering an environment where she feels understood and supported in navigating her stress and anxiety amidst cultural transition.

Case Study Simulation 2: Culturally Adapted MI for Managing Chronic Illness

Background: Juan is a 55-year-old man of Mexican descent who has recently been diagnosed with type 2 diabetes. He expresses frustration and resistance to changing his diet and lifestyle, which are closely tied to his cultural and family traditions. Juan is particularly concerned about not being able to participate in family meals and feeling isolated from his community due to his dietary restrictions.

Objective: As Juan's healthcare provider, using Motivational Interviewing (MI) adapted to respect and incorporate his cultural values, your goal is to help Juan explore his feelings about his diagnosis, enhance his motivation to manage his health effectively, and identify culturally appropriate strategies for adapting his diet and lifestyle.

Beginning of the Session

Healthcare Provider: "Juan, I appreciate you sharing your concerns with me today. Being diagnosed with diabetes can feel overwhelming, and I understand how important family meals and traditions are to you. Let's work together to find a way to manage your health that respects your cultural values. How does that sound to you?"

Expressing Empathy and Validating Feelings

Healthcare Provider: "It sounds like you're facing a tough situation, feeling caught between maintaining your health and staying connected to your cultural and family traditions. It's a difficult balance, and your feelings of frustration are completely valid. Let's explore this together."

Exploring Ambivalence

Healthcare Provider: "You mentioned feeling resistant to changing your diet because of its importance in your family and culture. Can you tell me more about what these traditions mean to you and how you feel about finding a balance between these traditions and your health needs?"

Reflecting Cultural Values in Goals

Healthcare Provider: "Family and community seem to play a significant role in your life, Juan. How can we use these values as a cornerstone to explore adjustments in your diet and lifestyle? Are there aspects of your traditions that might actually support your health goals?"

Addressing Cultural Mistrust and Barriers

Healthcare Provider: "I recognize that making these changes is not just a matter of willpower; it's about finding solutions that fit within your way of life. It's important that you feel understood and supported in this process. What are some concerns you have about adapting your lifestyle to manage your diabetes?"

Engaging with Cultural Strengths and Resources

Healthcare Provider: "Your cultural heritage includes a rich variety of foods and practices that can be beneficial for your health. Let's think creatively about how we can adapt traditional recipes and incorporate physical activities that you enjoy and that keep you connected to your community."

Planning for Change in a Culturally Sensitive Way

Healthcare Provider: "Considering the changes we've discussed, how do you feel about trying one small adjustment this week? For example, we could look at modifying a favorite family recipe to make it more diabetes-friendly while keeping the flavors you love."

Conclusion and Next Steps

Healthcare Provider: "Juan, I'm impressed by your willingness to explore these changes while honoring your traditions. Let's review your progress next time and adjust our plan as needed. Remember, this is a journey we're on together, and I'm here to support you every step of the way."

Summary

This case study highlights the importance of culturally sensitive MI in managing chronic illnesses like diabetes. By acknowledging Juan's cultural values and concerns, the healthcare provider creates a supportive space for Juan to explore his ambivalence, enhance his motivation for change, and identify culturally appropriate strategies for improving his health. This approach not only respects Juan's cultural identity but also empowers him to make sustainable lifestyle adjustments.

Chapter 9: Building Your MI Toolkit

Essential resources and tools for effective MI practice

Effective Motivational Interviewing (MI) practice requires a blend of knowledge, skills, and resources. Therapists and practitioners can enhance their MI techniques and outcomes by utilizing a variety of resources and tools designed to support both learning and application of MI principles. Here are essential resources and tools for effective MI practice:

1. Training Workshops and Certification Programs

- **Description:** Formal training programs, workshops, and certification courses offer comprehensive instruction in MI techniques, theory, and application. These programs often include live demonstrations, practice sessions, and feedback from experienced MI trainers.

- **Resource Example:** The Motivational Interviewing Network of Trainers (MINT) provides information on training opportunities, including introductory workshops and advanced training for MI practitioners seeking to deepen their skills.

2. Books and Manuals

- **Description:** Foundational texts and manuals authored by the creators of MI and other experts in the field serve as invaluable resources for understanding the nuances of MI and its application across different settings.

- **Resource Example:** "Motivational Interviewing: Helping People Change" by William R. Miller and Stephen Rollnick provides a comprehensive overview of MI principles, strategies, and applications.

3. Online Courses and Webinars

- **Description:** Online learning platforms offer accessible courses and webinars on MI, ranging from introductory overviews to topic-specific applications, such as MI in healthcare, addiction treatment, or mental health counseling.

- **Resource Example:** Platforms like Coursera, Udemy, and the American Psychological Association (APA) offer online courses and webinars taught by qualified instructors, allowing for flexible learning.

4. Supervision and Peer Consultation

- **Description:** Regular supervision or consultation with experienced MI practitioners provides opportunities for case discussion, feedback, and guidance on integrating MI into practice effectively.

- **Resource Example:** Establishing a relationship with an MI supervisor or joining a peer consultation group, possibly through professional networks or organizations like MINT, can enhance practical skills and therapeutic effectiveness.

5. Practice and Reflection Tools

- **Description:** Tools such as reflective journals, recording equipment for session review, and client feedback forms can aid in self-assessment and reflection on MI practice.

- **Resource Example:** Using a digital recorder to capture therapy sessions (with client consent) for later review and reflection, or employing apps designed for reflective practice and professional development.

6. Client Workbooks and Handouts

- **Description:** Workbooks and handouts designed for clients can supplement MI sessions by providing structured activities, reflection prompts, and educational materials that reinforce session content.

- **Resource Example:** Handouts on specific MI strategies, such as decisional balance exercises or values clarification activities, can support client engagement and motivation outside of sessions.

7. Research Journals and Articles

- **Description:** Staying informed about the latest research and developments in MI through scholarly journals and articles ensures that practice is grounded in the most current evidence.

- **Resource Example:** Journals such as the "Journal of Substance Abuse Treatment" or "Psychology of Addictive Behaviors" often publish articles on MI research, offering insights into its effectiveness and new applications.

8. Professional Networks and Organizations

- **Description:** Membership in professional networks or organizations dedicated to MI provides access to a community of practitioners, along with resources like newsletters, forums, and conferences.

- **Resource Example:** The Motivational Interviewing Network of Trainers (MINT) offers membership for MI practitioners, providing access to resources, networking opportunities, and updates on MI practice.

Conclusion

By leveraging these resources and tools, practitioners can continually refine their MI skills, stay abreast of the latest developments in the field, and provide the most effective support to their clients. Engaging with the broader MI community through training, supervision, and professional networks also fosters a culture of continuous learning and collaboration.

Apps and technology for enhancing MI skills

Incorporating apps and technology into Motivational Interviewing (MI) practice offers innovative ways to enhance skills, engage clients, and monitor progress. The digital landscape provides a wealth of resources for both practitioners and clients, supporting the principles of MI through interactive, accessible means. Here are several apps and technological tools that can augment MI skills and practice:

1. MI Skill-Building Apps

- **Examples:**

    - **MI Coach:** Designed for practitioners, this app offers scenarios, tips, and exercises to sharpen MI skills, including handling resistance, eliciting change talk, and strengthening commitment.

- **Practical MI:** Offers training modules and practice exercises to help therapists improve their MI techniques.

2. Video Role-Play Platforms

- **Examples:**

    - **SimSensei:** A platform that uses virtual avatars for role-playing therapeutic scenarios, allowing therapists to practice MI skills in a simulated environment.

    - **Rehearsal VRP (Virtual Role Play):** Offers a safe space for practitioners to practice MI conversations, receive feedback, and refine their approach based on AI-driven analysis.

3. Feedback and Reflection Tools

- **Examples:**

    - **Audio/Video Recording Software:** Apps like Audacity or simple smartphone video recording functions enable therapists to record practice sessions (with client consent) for self-review or supervision purposes, facilitating reflection on MI technique application.

    - **Reflectly:** While primarily a journaling app for clients, Reflectly can also be used by therapists to reflect on their practice, set professional development goals, and monitor progress in MI skills.

4. Educational and Training Resources

- Examples:

  - **Coursera and Udemy:** Online platforms offering courses on MI and related topics, taught by experts in the field. These courses can range from introductory overviews to advanced applications of MI in various contexts.

  - **Psychotherapy.net:** Provides video demonstrations of MI sessions by experts, serving as a valuable resource for observing and learning MI techniques.

5. Client Engagement and Monitoring Apps

- Examples:

  - **Motivational App:** Designed for client use, this app facilitates goal setting, tracks progress, and encourages reflection on motivations and barriers, aligning with MI's emphasis on client autonomy and motivation.

  - **Headspace:** While a mindfulness app, Headspace can support the MI process by helping clients engage with mindfulness practices to reduce ambivalence and enhance readiness for change.

6. Online Platforms for Secure Communication

- Examples:

  - **Zoom, Doxy.me, and other telehealth platforms:** These secure video conferencing tools are crucial for conducting remote MI sessions, ensuring privacy and accessibility while maintaining a high level of client engagement.

7. Digital Note-Taking and Organization Tools

- **Examples:**

    - **Evernote or Microsoft OneNote:** These apps can be used by therapists to organize notes, reflections, and resources related to MI practice, facilitating easy access to information and continuity of care.

Conclusion

The integration of apps and technology into MI practice not only enhances the skills of practitioners but also enriches the therapeutic experience for clients. By leveraging these digital resources, therapists can continue to grow their expertise, engage clients more effectively, and track progress in a structured, interactive manner. As technology evolves, so too will the opportunities to incorporate innovative tools into MI and other therapeutic practices.

Books, courses, and certifications for further learning.

Expanding your knowledge and skills in Motivational Interviewing (MI) and related areas can significantly enhance your practice and the outcomes for your clients. A combination of books, courses, and certification programs can provide a solid foundation for further learning. Here's a guide to some recommended resources:

Books

1. **"Motivational Interviewing: Helping People Change" (3rd Edition) by William R. Miller and Stephen Rollnick**

- This foundational text offers a comprehensive overview of MI principles and practices, written by the co-founders of MI.

2. **"Motivational Interviewing in Health Care: Helping Patients Change Behavior" by Stephen Rollnick, William R. Miller, and Christopher C. Butler**

   - Focuses on applying MI in healthcare settings, providing practical strategies for engaging patients and facilitating health-related behavior change.

3. **"Building Motivational Interviewing Skills: A Practitioner Workbook" by David B. Rosengren**

   - Offers a wealth of exercises and resources to practice and refine MI skills, suitable for both beginners and experienced practitioners.

Online Courses and Webinars

1. **Motivational Interviewing Network of Trainers (MINT)**

   - MINT offers resources for finding MI training and webinars led by certified MI trainers worldwide.

2. **Coursera**

   - Features courses on MI and related topics, such as "The Science of Well-Being" and "Psychological First Aid," which can complement MI practice by providing broader insights into behavior change and well-being.

3. **Psychotherapy.net**

- Provides video courses and demonstrations by leading practitioners in MI and other therapeutic approaches, offering insights into practical application and client interactions.

Certification Programs

1. **MINT Training for New Trainers (TNT)**

   - MINT offers an annual Training for New Trainers program, which is a key step for those seeking to become certified MI trainers. Completion of this program allows you to join MINT and access a community of MI practitioners and trainers.

2. **International Motivational Interviewing Network (IMIN) Certification**

   - IMIN offers a certification process for practitioners that involves demonstrating MI proficiency through recorded sessions and receiving feedback from certified reviewers.

3. **HealthSciences Institute**

   - Provides a "Certified Health Coach" program with a focus on MI, aimed at healthcare professionals looking to integrate coaching and MI into their practice.

Additional Resources

- **Local Workshops and Seminars:** Many professional associations and continuing education providers offer in-person and virtual workshops on MI. These can provide valuable hands-on experience and networking opportunities.

- **Peer Practice Groups:** Joining or forming a practice group with peers interested in MI can offer regular opportunities for practice, feedback, and mutual learning.

- **Research Journals:** Subscribing to journals that publish research on MI and behavior change can keep you updated on the latest findings and innovations in the field.

Conclusion

Whether you're new to MI or looking to deepen your expertise, a combination of reading foundational texts, engaging in structured learning through courses and webinars, and pursuing formal certification can significantly enhance your understanding and application of MI. Continuous learning and practice are key to mastering MI and effectively supporting your clients in their change processes.

Developing a personalized MI practice plan.

Developing a personalized Motivational Interviewing (MI) practice plan is a strategic approach to enhance your MI skills systematically. This plan should be tailored to your current level of expertise, learning style, and professional goals. Here's a step-by-step guide to creating an effective MI practice plan:

Step 1: Self-Assessment

- **Objective:** Evaluate your current MI skills and identify areas for improvement.

- **Action:** Use tools like the Motivational Interviewing Treatment Integrity (MITI) code to assess your proficiency. Reflect on feedback from clients, peers, and supervisors.

Step 2: Set Specific Goals

- **Objective:** Define clear, achievable goals based on your self-assessment.

- **Action:** Goals might include improving your reflective listening skills, using open-ended questions more effectively, or becoming proficient in rolling with resistance. Ensure goals are SMART (Specific, Measurable, Achievable, Relevant, Time-bound).

Step 3: Identify Learning Resources

- **Objective:** Compile a list of resources that align with your goals.

- **Action:** Choose from books, online courses, webinars, and workshops that focus on the areas you want to improve. Plan to join MI forums or networks for additional insights and support.

Step 4: Schedule Regular Practice

- **Objective:** Integrate MI practice into your daily routine.

- **Action:** Dedicate time in your schedule for role-playing exercises, reflecting on recorded sessions, or practicing MI techniques in real sessions. Consider practicing specific MI strategies with colleagues or in a peer practice group.

Step 5: Seek Feedback

- **Objective:** Obtain constructive feedback on your MI practice.

- **Action:** Arrange for peer or supervisor observations and feedback on your use of MI in sessions. Use client feedback forms to gauge how clients experience the MI approach with you.

Step 6: Reflect and Adjust

- **Objective:** Continuously evaluate your progress and adjust your plan as needed.

- **Action:** Regularly review your goals and the effectiveness of your learning activities. Reflect on what's working and what isn't, and be prepared to modify your plan to address new areas of growth.

Step 7: Professional Development

- **Objective:** Pursue formal training and certification to enhance your credibility and expertise.

- **Action:** Enroll in MI training programs or workshops offered by MINT or other reputable organizations. Consider working towards MI certification for professional development.

Step 8: Integrate Technology

- **Objective:** Leverage technology to support your MI practice.

- **Action:** Use apps and digital tools designed for MI training and client engagement. Explore platforms that offer virtual role-play and feedback opportunities.

Step 9: Cultivate Mindfulness

- **Objective:** Develop mindfulness skills to enhance presence and empathy in MI practice.

- **Action:** Incorporate mindfulness exercises into your daily routine to improve your ability to be present and attuned to clients during MI sessions.

Step 10: Community Engagement

- **Objective:** Engage with the MI community for support and continued learning.

- **Action:** Join MI forums, attend MI conferences, and participate in MINT activities. Sharing experiences and insights with fellow practitioners can provide motivation and fresh perspectives.

Step 11: Document Progress

- **Objective:** Keep a detailed record of your MI practice and progress.

- **Action:** Maintain a professional journal to document your experiences, reflections, and insights gained from practicing MI. Note specific instances where MI techniques were particularly effective or challenging, and reflect on client outcomes related to these instances.

Step 12: Incorporate Cultural Competence

- **Objective:** Enhance your ability to apply MI in a culturally sensitive manner.

- **Action:** Seek out resources and training on cultural competence in MI. Actively apply these learnings by tailoring MI approaches to respect and incorporate the cultural backgrounds and values of your clients.

Step 13: Expand Your MI Application

- **Objective:** Broaden the application of MI beyond its traditional contexts.

- **Action:** Experiment with applying MI principles in a variety of settings or with different client populations. For example, explore how MI can be adapted for group therapy sessions, telehealth, or clients with co-occurring disorders.

Step 14: Participate in MI Research

- **Objective:** Contribute to the MI body of knowledge and stay informed about the latest research findings.

- **Action:** Engage with ongoing MI research, either by participating in studies, applying research findings to your practice, or attending presentations and readings on new MI research. Consider conducting your own research to explore the effectiveness of MI interventions in specific contexts or populations.

Step 15: Mentorship and Training Others

- **Objective:** Share your MI knowledge and skills with others.

- **Action:** As you become more proficient in MI, consider mentoring less experienced practitioners or offering training sessions. Sharing your knowledge can reinforce your own skills and provide valuable support to the professional community.

Continuous Improvement Cycle

- **Objective:** Maintain a cycle of continuous improvement in your MI practice.

- **Action:** Regularly return to Step 1 to reassess your skills and goals. The field of MI, like all areas of psychotherapy, is dynamic, with new insights and techniques continually emerging. Staying engaged with the process of self-assessment and goal-setting ensures that your practice remains current and effective.

Example of a Personalized MI Practice Plan

- **Goal:** Improve the use of complex reflections in sessions.

- **Resources:** "Building Motivational Interviewing Skills: A Practitioner Workbook" by David B. Rosengren; enroll in an online course on advanced MI techniques.

- **Practice:** Dedicate 15 minutes daily to role-playing exercises focusing on complex reflections; use one session per week to specifically focus on this skill.

- **Feedback:** Monthly review sessions with a supervisor to discuss progress and challenges; use client feedback forms to assess the impact of enhanced reflective listening skills.

- **Adjustment:** Based on feedback, incorporate new strategies or focus on additional areas, such as eliciting change talk more effectively.

By following these steps and regularly reviewing and adjusting your plan, you can create a dynamic and effective pathway to mastering Motivational Interviewing, tailored to your unique professional journey and goals.

Chapter 10: The Future of Motivational Interviewing

Emerging trends and research in MI

Emerging trends and research in Motivational Interviewing (MI) are shaping the way this therapeutic approach is applied and understood in various contexts. These developments reflect the dynamic and adaptable nature of MI, as researchers and practitioners explore its applications beyond traditional settings, integrate technology, and focus on specific populations or issues. Here are some key emerging trends and research areas in MI:

1. Digital MI Applications

- **Trend:** The use of digital platforms and mobile applications to deliver MI interventions is growing. These technologies offer new ways to reach and engage clients, providing flexibility and accessibility that traditional face-to-face sessions cannot.

- **Research Focus:** Studies are examining the effectiveness of digital MI interventions, exploring how aspects like personalized feedback, interactive modules, and text messaging support can enhance motivation and engagement in behavior change.

2. Integration with Other Therapeutic Approaches

- **Trend:** There is increasing interest in how MI can be integrated with other evidence-based therapies, such as Cognitive Behavioral Therapy (CBT), Dialectical Behavior

Therapy (DBT), and Acceptance and Commitment Therapy (ACT), to enhance treatment outcomes.

- **Research Focus:** Research is exploring the synergistic effects of combining MI with other therapies, particularly in treating complex issues like substance abuse, eating disorders, and dual diagnoses.

3. Precision MI

- **Trend:** Precision MI refers to the tailoring of MI interventions to the individual characteristics, preferences, and cultural backgrounds of clients. This approach recognizes the diversity of clients and seeks to optimize MI's effectiveness by personalizing its application.

- **Research Focus:** Studies are investigating how factors such as cultural background, gender, age, and specific psychological needs influence the effectiveness of MI and how MI can be adapted to better meet these diverse needs.

4. MI in Public Health and Policy

- **Trend:** MI is being applied more broadly in public health initiatives and policy-making to address societal issues such as smoking cessation, obesity, and vaccination hesitancy. This reflects a shift towards using MI to influence behavior change on a larger scale.

- **Research Focus:** Research is evaluating the impact of MI-based interventions in public health campaigns, policy development, and community programs, looking at outcomes like increased engagement, behavior change, and public health improvements.

5. Mechanisms of Change in MI

- **Trend:** There is a deepening investigation into the mechanisms through which MI facilitates behavior change. Understanding these mechanisms can enhance the effectiveness of MI by refining how it is taught and practiced.

- **Research Focus:** Research is delving into aspects such as the role of client autonomy, the therapeutic relationship, specific MI techniques (like reflective listening and change talk), and how these elements contribute to successful outcomes.

6. Training and Fidelity

- **Trend:** As MI continues to evolve, there is an ongoing focus on how practitioners are trained in MI techniques and how fidelity to the MI model is maintained in diverse settings.

- **Research Focus:** Studies are examining the most effective training methods for MI, including online training, supervision, feedback mechanisms, and the role of ongoing professional development in maintaining high-quality MI practice.

7. Special Populations

- **Trend:** The application of MI is expanding to special populations, such as children and adolescents, the elderly, and individuals with specific health conditions or cultural backgrounds.

- **Research Focus:** Research is exploring the adaptations required to effectively apply MI with these groups, focusing

178

on age-appropriate communication, cultural sensitivity, and addressing unique challenges faced by these populations.

These emerging trends and research areas underscore the versatility and potential of MI to contribute to various fields of practice and research. As evidence continues to accumulate, MI is likely to remain at the forefront of interventions aimed at promoting positive behavior change.

Artificial intelligence and machine learning in MI training

The role of artificial intelligence (AI) and machine learning (ML) in Motivational Interviewing (MI) training is an exciting and rapidly evolving area. These technologies are beginning to transform how MI training is delivered, personalized, and scaled, offering innovative ways to enhance the skills of practitioners. Here are some key aspects of how AI and ML contribute to MI training:

1. Simulation and Virtual Training Environments

- AI can create realistic, interactive simulations or virtual environments where practitioners can practice MI techniques without the need for real-life interactions initially. These simulations can mimic a wide range of client scenarios and personalities, offering practitioners a safe space to practice and refine their skills.

- Virtual clients powered by AI can provide real-time feedback to the practitioners based on their responses, enabling immediate learning and adjustment.

2. Personalized Learning

- Machine learning algorithms can analyze a practitioner's performance in training simulations to identify strengths and areas for improvement. Based on this analysis, the AI can tailor the training content to address specific skill gaps, ensuring a more personalized learning experience.

- Personalized feedback mechanisms can highlight specific areas where a practitioner might need to focus more, such as improving reflective listening skills or better handling resistance.

3. Automated Assessment and Feedback

- AI can be used to assess MI fidelity and competence by analyzing recorded training sessions. Natural language processing (NLP) and machine learning algorithms can evaluate the use of MI techniques, the quality of the therapeutic conversation, and adherence to the MI spirit.

- Automated feedback can provide practitioners with objective, detailed insights into their MI practice, identifying specific moments in the conversation where improvements could be made.

4. Scalability and Accessibility

- AI and ML technologies make it possible to scale MI training to a larger number of practitioners without the need for extensive human resources. This is particularly beneficial for organizations and regions with limited access to MI trainers.

- Online platforms powered by AI can offer accessible MI training opportunities, breaking down geographical and logistical barriers and enabling continuous learning.

5. Ongoing Learning and Skill Enhancement

- AI-driven platforms can support ongoing learning and skill enhancement by offering regular, easy-to-access training exercises, updates on best practices, and insights into the latest MI research.

- Continuous learning environments can help practitioners stay engaged with MI principles and techniques, fostering a culture of professional development and excellence.

6. Data-Driven Insights for Training Improvement

- By collecting and analyzing data from training sessions, AI and ML can provide valuable insights into common challenges faced by practitioners, effectiveness of different training modules, and overall trends in MI training outcomes.

- These insights can inform the development of future training programs, ensuring they are evidence-based and aligned with practitioners' needs.

The integration of AI and ML in MI training represents a promising frontier for enhancing the effectiveness and reach of MI education. As these technologies continue to advance, they are likely to play an increasingly significant role in shaping the future of MI training, making it more personalized, efficient, and impactful.

Envisioning the future of MI in mental health care.

Envisioning the future of Motivational Interviewing (MI) in mental health care involves recognizing its evolving role amidst technological advancements, shifting healthcare landscapes, and a growing understanding of its application across diverse populations and settings. As we look ahead, several key trends and possibilities emerge, shaping how MI will continue to contribute to mental health care:

1. Wider Integration Across Health Disciplines

MI's principles and techniques, rooted in promoting behavior change through empathy and understanding, will likely see broader application beyond traditional mental health settings. We can expect its integration into primary care, chronic disease management, substance abuse treatment, and public health initiatives, emphasizing its role in a holistic approach to health and wellbeing.

2. Enhanced Training and Accessibility

With advancements in technology, particularly artificial intelligence (AI) and virtual reality (VR), the training for MI will become more interactive, accessible, and personalized. These technologies will enable scalable training solutions, making MI skills more accessible to healthcare professionals globally. This democratization of MI training can lead to a more widespread adoption of MI techniques across various healthcare sectors.

3. Digital Therapeutics and Telehealth

The future of MI in mental health care will be significantly influenced by the expansion of digital therapeutics and telehealth. MI techniques will be adapted for digital platforms, allowing practitioners to engage with clients through online counseling sessions, mobile apps, and other digital health tools. This will not only extend the reach of MI to underserved populations but also integrate MI into digital health interventions, enhancing their effectiveness and engagement.

4. Personalized and Precision Medicine

As the medical field moves towards more personalized and precision-based approaches, MI's flexibility and client-centered nature make it an ideal complement. MI can be tailored to fit the individual's unique motivations, challenges, and goals, aligning with the broader shift towards personalized care plans that consider genetic, environmental, and lifestyle factors.

5. Cross-Cultural Adaptation and Inclusivity

There will be a growing emphasis on adapting MI to be culturally sensitive and inclusive, ensuring it is effective across diverse populations. Research and practice will focus on understanding how MI can be modified to respect cultural norms, values, and communication styles, making it a more universally applicable tool for behavior change.

6. Collaboration with Emerging Therapeutic Approaches

MI's future in mental health care will also see increased collaboration with emerging therapeutic approaches, such as mindfulness-based interventions, digital CBT (cognitive behavioral therapy), and DBT (dialectical behavior therapy). Integrating MI with these therapies can enhance their effectiveness, offering a more comprehensive approach to treatment that leverages the strengths of each methodology.

7. Outcome Measurement and Evidence-Based Practice

Advancements in data analytics and outcome measurement tools will enable more sophisticated assessments of MI's effectiveness in various contexts. This will support the ongoing refinement of MI techniques and their application, ensuring that practice is driven by evidence and results in improved client outcomes.

8. Policy and Systemic Change

Finally, as the evidence base for MI's effectiveness in promoting health and wellbeing continues to grow, there may be increased advocacy for incorporating MI principles into health policy and systemic approaches to care. This could involve training healthcare professionals in MI as a standard part of their education, incorporating MI into public health campaigns, and using MI to inform patient engagement and health promotion strategies at the systemic level.

Envisioning the future of MI in mental health care is to anticipate a dynamic and expanding role for this therapeutic approach, driven by innovation, inclusivity, and an unwavering commitment to supporting individuals in their journey towards better health and wellbeing.

Appendices

Glossary of MI Terms

Creating a glossary of Motivational Interviewing (MI) terms helps clarify key concepts, techniques, and principles integral to the practice. Here's a concise glossary:

1. Motivational Interviewing (MI)

A client-centered, directive method for enhancing intrinsic motivation to change by exploring and resolving ambivalence.

2. Ambivalence

Mixed feelings or simultaneous conflicting attitudes toward a particular behavior change. In MI, ambivalence is viewed as a natural part of the change process.

3. Change Talk

Statements made by clients expressing desire, ability, reasons, or need for change. MI techniques aim to elicit and reinforce change talk as a pathway to behavior change.

4. Resistance (or Sustain Talk)

Statements by clients expressing reluctance to change, often viewed as an indication of the therapist's approach being misaligned with the client's readiness for change. MI seeks to respond to resistance in a way that respects the client's autonomy and perspectives.

5. OARS

An acronym for the foundational MI skills:

- **Open-ended questions**

- **Affirmations**

- **Reflective listening**

- **Summaries**

6. Reflective Listening

A key MI skill where the therapist listens attentively to the client and then reflects back the essence of what the client has said, often with a new perspective or emphasis, to deepen understanding or elicit change talk.

7. Empathy

A core principle of MI, involving a deep, nonjudgmental, compassionate understanding of the client's perspective and feelings.

8. Rolling with Resistance

An MI strategy that involves accepting and validating the client's feelings and perspectives without direct confrontation, aiming to decrease resistance and explore new viewpoints.

9. Decisional Balance

An exercise used in MI to explore the pros and cons of changing versus not changing a behavior, aimed at clarifying the client's values and motivations.

10. Discrepancy

Highlighting the gap between a client's current behavior and broader goals or values to enhance motivation for change.

11. Self-Efficacy

A person's belief in their ability to succeed in specific situations or accomplish a task. MI aims to boost self-efficacy regarding behavior change.

12. Readiness to Change

A client's current stage in the process of changing a particular behavior. MI recognizes different stages of readiness and seeks to match intervention strategies accordingly.

13. MI Spirit

The underlying ethos of MI, characterized by collaboration (vs. confrontation), evocation (vs. education), and autonomy (vs. authority), emphasizing respect for the client's autonomy and fostering a partnership.

14. SMART Goals

Specific, Measurable, Achievable, Relevant, and Time-bound objectives set in collaboration with the client to facilitate concrete steps towards behavior change.

15. Complex Reflection

An MI technique where the therapist makes a guess about the underlying meaning of what the client has said, often leading to deeper exploration or insight.

This glossary covers fundamental MI terms that are crucial for understanding and applying the approach effectively in various therapeutic contexts.

16. Coding

In the context of MI, coding refers to the process of reviewing and evaluating segments of therapy sessions to assess fidelity to MI principles, including how well the therapist adheres to the techniques and spirit of MI.

17. Elicit-Provide-Elicit

A technique in MI for providing information or advice. First, the therapist elicits the client's knowledge or needs regarding a topic, then provides information in a permission-based manner, and finally elicits the client's response to the information provided.

18. Menu of Options

Offering a client a range of choices or strategies for change, respecting their autonomy and empowering them to choose the path that feels most suitable for them.

19. Normalization

A technique used in MI to reassure clients that their experiences or feelings are common and understandable, reducing feelings of isolation or shame.

20. Preparatory Change Talk

Statements by clients indicating consideration of, but not full commitment to change, including expressions of desire, ability, reasons, and need for change.

21. Mobilizing Change Talk

Statements by clients that indicate a commitment to change, including expressions of commitment, activation, and taking steps toward change.

22. Sustain Talk

Expressions from the client that argue against change, highlighting the client's desire to maintain the status quo. It's distinct from resistance in that it directly relates to the target behavior rather than the therapeutic process.

23. Therapeutic Paradox

An MI technique where the therapist intentionally exaggerates the argument against change, aiming to elicit from the client arguments in favor of change, often used carefully to navigate resistance.

24. Values Clarification

An MI strategy that involves exploring what is most important to the client, to enhance motivation for change by linking desired changes to the client's core values.

25. Motivational Discrepancy

Creating awareness in clients about the discrepancy between their current behavior and their broader life values or goals, which can motivate them towards change.

26. Process Questions

Questions asked by the therapist to help clients reflect on their own change process, enhancing their awareness of the stages of change and facilitating movement towards action.

27. Strengths-Based Approach

Focusing on and leveraging the client's existing strengths and successes as a foundation for fostering change, rather than concentrating solely on problems or deficits.

28. Feedback Loop

A method in MI involving giving clients specific feedback about their behavior and its consequences, designed to increase their awareness and prompt contemplation about change.

29. Commitment Language

Statements by the client that signal a strong commitment to change, seen as predictive of actual changes in behavior. Therapists aim to elicit and reinforce this language.

30. MI-Consistent Responses

Responses from the therapist that align with the spirit of MI, including empathy, support for autonomy, collaboration, and evocation of the client's own motivations for change.

Frequently Asked Questions (FAQs) about MI.

Frequently Asked Questions (FAQs) about Motivational Interviewing (MI)

1. What is Motivational Interviewing?

Motivational Interviewing (MI) is a collaborative, goal-oriented style of communication with particular attention to the language of change. It is designed to strengthen personal motivation for and commitment to a specific goal by eliciting and exploring the person's own reasons for change within an atmosphere of acceptance and compassion.

2. Who can benefit from MI?

MI can benefit a wide range of individuals across various settings, including healthcare, mental health, addiction treatment, counseling, and more. It's particularly useful for individuals who are ambivalent or resistant to change.

3. How does MI differ from other therapeutic approaches?

MI is distinct in its focus on collaboration rather than confrontation, evoking rather than educating, and autonomy rather than authority. It emphasizes the client's own motivation and commitment to change, rather than the therapist's agenda.

4. Can MI be integrated with other therapies?

Yes, MI can be effectively integrated with other therapeutic approaches, such as Cognitive Behavioral Therapy (CBT) and Dialectical Behavior Therapy (DBT), to enhance the overall therapeutic process and outcomes.

5. How long does MI take to show results?

The timeline for seeing results from MI varies depending on the individual and their context. Some clients may experience significant shifts in motivation and begin making changes after just one or two sessions, while others may require more time.

6. Is MI evidence-based?

Yes, MI is supported by a substantial body of research indicating its effectiveness in promoting behavior change across a variety of issues, including substance abuse, health behavior changes, and mental health conditions.

7. What are the core principles of MI?

The core principles of MI include expressing empathy, developing discrepancy, rolling with resistance, and supporting self-efficacy.

8. How is success measured in MI?

Success in MI can be measured through various outcomes, including increased motivation for change, resolution of ambivalence, concrete steps taken towards change, and achievement of specific goals.

9. Can MI be used in group settings?

Yes, MI can be adapted for use in group settings, where it can facilitate collective motivation and support for change among participants.

10. **How can I learn MI?**

Learning MI typically involves attending workshops, training sessions, and engaging in practice with feedback. It is also helpful to study MI through books, online courses, and supervision from experienced practitioners.

11. **Is MI culturally sensitive?**

MI is designed to be flexible and adaptable, making it suitable for application across different cultures. Its emphasis on respect for the individual and their values supports cultural sensitivity and competence.

12. **Can MI be delivered through telehealth?**

Yes, MI can be effectively delivered through telehealth platforms, allowing for the continuation of therapy and support remotely.

13. **What are the challenges of using MI?**

Practitioners may face challenges such as mastering the technique, staying patient-centered, and effectively managing their own reactions to clients' resistance or ambivalence.

14. **How does MI handle resistance?**

MI approaches resistance not as opposition to be overcome but as a signal for the therapist to adjust their approach, focusing on building rapport and exploring the underlying causes of the resistance.

15. How do therapists develop competence in MI?

Developing competence in MI involves a combination of formal training, ongoing practice, receiving feedback from skilled practitioners, and self-reflection. Many therapists also engage in peer practice groups or seek certification through recognized MI training organizations.

16. Can MI be used with children and adolescents?

Yes, MI has been adapted for use with children and adolescents, particularly in addressing behavioral issues, substance use, and promoting health-related behaviors. It requires adjustments in approach to suit the developmental stage of the young client.

17. What role does empathy play in MI?

Empathy is a cornerstone of MI, as it creates a safe and supportive environment for clients to explore their ambivalence and motivations for change. Showing genuine understanding and acceptance is crucial to fostering a productive therapeutic relationship.

18. How does MI handle clients who are not ready to change?

MI is particularly effective with clients who are ambivalent or not yet ready to change. It respects the client's autonomy and pace, gently exploring the pros and cons of change without pushing them to make a decision before they are ready.

19. What are some common misconceptions about MI?

Some misconceptions include the idea that MI is only for substance abuse problems, that it's simply a way of being nice to clients, or that it doesn't require structured training to practice effectively.

These misunderstandings overlook the strategic and skillful nature of MI.

20. Can MI be used for self-help?

While MI is primarily a therapeutic technique delivered by a trained practitioner, the principles of MI can inform self-help strategies, such as self-reflection on ambivalence, exploring personal motivations for change, and setting goals.

21. How does MI view relapse or setbacks?

In MI, relapse or setbacks are viewed as part of the change process rather than failures. These experiences are opportunities for learning and growth, and MI helps clients to explore what can be learned from these situations to aid future attempts at change.

22. Can MI be applied in non-clinical settings?

Yes, MI has been successfully applied in a variety of non-clinical settings, including education, sports coaching, business management, and public health interventions, to encourage positive behavioral changes.

23. How does MI align with ethical standards in therapy?

MI aligns well with ethical standards in therapy by promoting respect for client autonomy, non-coercion, beneficence (acting in the best interest of the client), and nonmaleficence (avoiding harm to the client).

24. What is the future of MI?

The future of MI includes its continued integration with technology, expansion in its application across various disciplines and cultures, and ongoing research to refine its techniques and understand its effectiveness in new areas.

25. **How can clients prepare for MI therapy?**

Clients can prepare for MI therapy by reflecting on their feelings about change, considering their goals, and being open to exploring their ambivalence in a supportive environment. Being prepared to engage actively in the process can enhance the effectiveness of MI.

These FAQs cover some of the most common inquiries about Motivational Interviewing, providing a foundational understanding for those interested in learning more about this approach to facilitating change.

Directory of MI Resources and Organizations

To further explore and engage with Motivational Interviewing (MI), various resources and organizations offer in-depth information, training, and community support. Here's a directory to help you navigate these options:

1. **Motivational Interviewing Network of Trainers (MINT)**

- **Description**: An international organization committed to promoting high-quality MI practice and training. Offers resources, a directory of trainers, and information on becoming a member.

- **Website**: <u>Motivational Interviewing Network of Trainers (MINT)</u>

2. **The International Journal of Behavioral Consultation and Therapy (IJBCT)**

- **Description**: Publishes research related to MI and its applications across different fields. A valuable resource for staying updated on the latest MI research and practice developments.

- **Website**: IJBCT

3. The Center for Motivation and Change (CMC)

- **Description**: Offers training in MI and other evidence-based approaches for professionals, as well as resources for individuals and families looking to understand and implement change.

- **Website**: The Center for Motivation and Change

4. Addiction Technology Transfer Center (ATTC) Network

- **Description**: Focuses on enhancing clinical practice related to addiction treatment and recovery services, including MI training opportunities.

- **Website**: ATTC Network

5. Society of Clinical Psychology (Division 12 of APA)

- **Description**: Offers resources on evidence-based practices in psychology, including MI. A good source for professionals seeking to integrate MI with other therapeutic approaches.

- **Website**: Society of Clinical Psychology

6. The Guilford Press

- **Description**: Publishes seminal books on MI, including works by MI founders Miller and Rollnick, providing essential reading for practitioners at all levels.

- **Website**: The Guilford Press

7. Psychwire

- **Description**: Offers online courses on MI and other psychological approaches, taught by leading experts in the field. A convenient way to learn MI skills online.

- **Website**: Psychwire

8. MI Trainers' Resources

- **Description**: A hub for MI trainers to share tools, exercises, and training materials. Great for trainers seeking to enrich their MI training sessions.

- **Website**: Typically accessed through MINT and other professional networks.

9. MI Chatbots and Apps

- **Description**: Various digital tools and apps are available to practice MI skills, receive training, and support clients in making changes. Examples include "Change Talk" and "Motivate Me."

- **Website**: Available on app stores and specific product websites.

10. MI Training Workshops and Conferences

- **Description**: Regular workshops, seminars, and conferences are held globally, offering opportunities for direct training, networking, and professional development in MI.

- **Website**: Information available through MINT, local psychological associations, and continuing education providers.

This directory serves as a starting point for exploring the wealth of resources and organizations dedicated to Motivational Interviewing. Whether you're a practitioner looking to deepen your MI skills, a researcher interested in the latest findings, or someone interested in applying MI principles in your life or work, these resources offer valuable insights and opportunities for engagement.

References

1. **Miller, W.R., & Rollnick, S. (2013).** *Motivational Interviewing: Helping People Change*. Guilford Press. This foundational text by the creators of MI provides comprehensive insights into the principles, processes, and practicalities of MI.

2. **Arkowitz, H., Miller, W.R., & Rollnick, S. (Eds.). (2015).** *Motivational Interviewing in the Treatment of Psychological Problems*. Guilford Press. This book explores the application of MI across a range of psychological issues, offering case studies and clinical strategies.

3. **Hettema, J., Steele, J., & Miller, W.R. (2005).** *Motivational Interviewing.* Annual Review of Clinical Psychology, 1, 91-111. This review offers a concise overview of MI's theoretical underpinnings and its efficacy in promoting behavior change.

4. **Moyers, T.B., Martin, T., Manuel, J.K., Miller, W.R., & Ernst, D. (2010).** *Revised Global Scales: Motivational Interviewing Treatment Integrity 3.1.1 (MITI 3.1.1).* University of New Mexico, Center on Alcoholism, Substance Abuse, and Addictions (CASAA). The MITI scales provide a framework for assessing MI fidelity and effectiveness in clinical settings.

5. **Rollnick, S., Miller, W.R., & Butler, C.C. (2008).** *Motivational Interviewing in Health Care: Helping Patients Change Behavior*. Guilford Press. This book discusses the application of MI within healthcare settings, emphasizing patient-centered care and behavior change in patients.

6. **Wagner, C.C., & Ingersoll, K.S. (2013).** *Motivational Interviewing in Groups.* Guilford Press. Offering insights into using MI in group settings, this reference expands on the adaptability and application of MI principles beyond individual therapy.

7. **Smedslund, G., Berg, R.C., Hammerstrøm, K.T., Steiro, A., Leiknes, K.A., Dahl, H.M., & Karlsen, K. (2011).** *Motivational interviewing for substance abuse.* Cochrane Database of Systematic Reviews, Issue 5. Art. No.: CD008063. This systematic review evaluates the effectiveness of MI in treating substance abuse, providing evidence-based insights into its efficacy.

8. **Lundahl, B., & Burke, B.L. (2009).** *The effectiveness and applicability of motivational interviewing: A practice-friendly review of four meta-analyses.* Journal of Clinical Psychology, 65(11), 1232-1245. This article reviews the evidence supporting MI's effectiveness, making a case for its broad applicability in clinical practice.

9. **Madson, M.B., & Campbell, T.C. (2006).** *Measures of fidelity in motivational enhancement: A systematic review.* Journal of Substance Abuse Treatment, 31(1), 67-73. Focusing on the measurement of MI fidelity, this review highlights the importance of adherence to MI principles for effective practice.

10. **Rosengren, D.B. (2009).** *Building Motivational Interviewing Skills: A Practitioner Workbook.* Guilford Press. A practical workbook that offers exercises and strategies for clinicians looking to build and refine their MI skills.